Adolescents and Substance Use

The handbook for professionals working with young people

South London and Maudsley NHS Trust
Honorary Senior Lecturer, Institute of Psychiatry, King's College London
Founder, Global Drugs Service

Radcliffe Publishing
London • New York

Radcliffe Publishing Ltd
St Mark's House
Shepherdess Walk
London N1 7LH
United Kingdom

www.radcliffehealth.com

British Library Cataloguing in Publication Data

A catalogue record for this book is available from the British Library.

ISBN-13: 978 184619 979 0

The paper used for the text pages of this book is FSC® certified. FSC (The Forest Stewardship Council®) is an international network to promote responsible management of the world's forests.

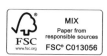

Typeset by Beautiful Words, Auckland, New Zealand
Printed and bound by TJI Digital, Padstow, Cornwall, UK

Contents

Foreword

When I was asked to write the foreword for this book my first thought was to question whether the world needed another book on drug and alcohol use. Then I looked more carefully at the title and noticed a rather important word – 'adolescents'. I then reconsidered and reflected on my own practice with mainly adults and remembered how I often complained that so little was ever done earlier in their lives to alter the trajectory of their substance use. It is a failing of our treatment system that we seem to wait for people to develop entrenched substance use problems and accompanying criminal records before we consider providing treatment. Indeed it is perverse that across so many of our health, social and educational systems we invest a disproportionate amount in the later years of life, where the potential gains, compared to early life investment, are diminishingly slim. You can see where this is leading I assume?

This book is an important addition to libraries on substance use because it provides the professions and people who often have first access to individuals at risk of developing substance use problems with the background knowledge and framework for skills development to intervene and make a difference.

Clearly written by likeable clinical experts in their fields from across the social and medical disciplines, this book takes the informed or novice reader on an enlightening journey through developmental functional neuroanatomy (not scary at all thanks to the way they write about it) and its susceptibility to drug-related harm and the often ignored issues of protective factors and the role of the family.

While the areas on prevention, mental illness and motivational interviewing are stock content for any book, the chapters here are written concisely with enough theoretical grounding and evidence to convince the reader but without redundant stuffing stating the obvious. Chapters on culture, sexuality, policy and ethical issues are often poorly addressed, even in the adult literature, so finding them is a welcome surprise.

As the English-speaking world wakes up to the challenge of novel psycho-active substances and the grinding weight of research slowly leads to change in policy and how we communicate with people in our communities, a book about young people and drugs is timely. If we could delay the onset of drug use in our most vulnerable young people and promote the acquisition of skills among young people so that they could grow their brains before they tried to expand them with drugs, we could make a real difference. This book, by helping diverse health and social professionals to recognise when substance use may be diminishing the potential and wellbeing of a person, could therefore play an important role in helping our communities to be happier healthier places for everyone.

Dr Adam R Winstock
MD, MRCP, MRCPsych, FAChAM
Consultant Psychiatrist and Addiction Medicine Specialist
South London and Maudsley NHS Trust
Honorary Senior Lecturer, Institute of Psychiatry, King's College London
September 2013

Preface

In our work with adolescents with substance use problems we have collaborated with a variety of professionals who also engage with these young people and their families. An exhaustive list is impossible, but it includes social workers, social care professionals, family support workers, teachers, counsellors, mental health teams, accident and emergency staff, as well as the police and probation officers. They have often asked us to recommend a book that provides an introduction to adolescent substance use. These professionals, while not substance abuse practitioners, invariably come to work with teenagers with drug and alcohol problems. Unfortunately, we could not identify a book that filled this gap. Slowly it dawned on us that if such a book was to be written, we might have to write it ourselves. So in the summer of 2011, the idea for this book began to germinate. We spoke to and elicited email feedback from various colleagues about what such a book ought to include, and gradually the book took shape.

The aim of this book is to provide an introduction to the topic of adolescent substance use and, ideally, guidance for the numerous professionals who work with teenagers. It is difficult to imagine that any professional who works with teenagers will not come across substance use at some point. The approach these practitioners take in dealing with the problem has considerable influence over the outcome, and so this book hopes to provide a foundation for effective, evidence-based practice.

PJ, CK, AC, BPS
September 2013

About the authors

Philip James, MSc, BSc (Hons), RPN, Dip Psych Nurs, MAREBT
Philip trained as a psychiatric nurse in Dublin and was appointed as the first Irish Clinical Nurse Specialist in Adolescent Substance Misuse in 2006. Since then he has worked in the Health Service Executive's Youth Drug and Alcohol (YoDA) Service full-time. He completed a MSc in nursing in 2005 and is also qualified in Rational Emotive Behaviour Therapy and the Adolescent Community Reinforcement Approach. In addition to his clinical work he has been involved in a number of research projects and publications. He has published various research articles and, along with Bobby Smyth, contributed a chapter to *Responding in Mental Health – Substance Use* (2011), also published by Radcliffe. He is a reviewer for various international academic journals and is on the International Advisory Committee of the journal *Mental Health and Substance Use*. He has provided lectures on a variety of addiction, mental health and practice-related topics with a number of colleges, including University College Dublin, Trinity College Dublin, the University of Limerick, the Institute of Integrative Counselling and Psychotherapy and the Irish College of Humanities and Applied Sciences.

Caitríona Kearns, BSc (Hons), MIACP, MWGII
Caitríona is the General Manager and Registrar of the Institute of Integrative Counselling and Psychotherapy, and the Clinical Manager of the Village Counselling Service, a community counselling charity in Dublin, Ireland. She is an accredited member of the Irish Association for Counselling and Psychotherapy. Caitríona obtained her addiction counselling qualifications in the International Addiction Counsellor Training Programme, a Hazelden-endorsed programme. Her BSc in counselling and psychotherapy was conferred by Middlesex University. Prior to her current role, she spent 10 years working in the field of substance misuse treatment, specialising in counselling children and adolescents. At present, Caitríona lectures on the Institute of Integrative Counselling and Psychotherapy's BA (Hons) in counselling and psychotherapy,

leading the modules on addiction and sexuality and overseeing the clinical aspects of students' development.

Ann Campbell, MSc, RGN, Dip Addct St, Dip Syst Psych
Member Family Therapy Association of Ireland and the Irish Council for Psychotherapy

Ann works with adolescents, parents and families who are experiencing problems with drug and alcohol use, as a Systemic Family Psychotherapist in the Youth Drug and Alcohol (YoDA) Service in Dublin. She completed the Diploma in Addiction Studies and the MSc in Child Adolescent and Family Mental Health in Trinity College, Dublin; including a work placement in Turning Point, Melbourne, Australia. Ann has worked in addiction and family support services since 1997, initially in a nursing role. Her interaction with adults making changes with substance misuse prompted her interest in systemic perspectives; she began Systemic Psychotherapy training at the Clanwilliam Institute in 1999. Ann has worked with adolescents and families through the Crinan Youth Project, West Dublin YMCA PAKT (Parents and Kids Together) family support project and joined YoDA in 2007.

Ann has particular interests in research, narrative therapy and parents' perspectives in adolescent substance misuse. She has investigated adolescent use of novel psychoactive substances, presenting at the Association of Child and Adolescent Mental Health Conference and the Irish National Drugs Conference. Ann has facilitated workshops in family therapy, inter-agency working and adolescent drug misuse. Currently Ann is vice-chairperson of the Family Therapy Association of Ireland.

Dr Bobby P Smyth, MRCPsych, MB BCh BAO

Dr Bobby P Smyth is a Consultant Child and Adolescent Psychiatrist, working full-time since 2003 with adolescents who have substance use disorders. He is clinical lead at three separate multidisciplinary outpatient treatment services for adolescents with substance use problems. He also consults to a residential adolescent drug and alcohol treatment programme. He graduated in medicine from University College Dublin in Ireland. He completed his basic specialist training in psychiatry in Dublin before undertaking higher specialist training in child and adolescent psychiatry in Liverpool and Chester, UK. He was a member of the Executive Committee of the Child and Adolescent Psychiatry faculty of the Royal College of Psychiatrists.

He is also a Clinical Associate Professor with the Department of Public Health and Primary Care in Trinity College Dublin. He has been involved in addiction research since 1993 and has published over 50 addiction research papers in national and international peer-reviewed journals on topics including treatment outcome, harms associated with drug abuse and early-onset drinking. He has presented at numerous international scientific meetings. This research has spanned diverse areas of science from neurobiology to sociology and psychology. His research has won prizes from the Royal College of Psychiatrists (UK) and the Royal Academy of Medicine of Ireland.

He has been a member of a number of national policy committees on alcohol and drugs in Ireland. He has been invited to present to committees of elected representatives on policy issues regarding alcohol and drugs. He features regularly on television, radio and print media on topics related to substance use. He is a member of the National Addiction Training Programme in Ireland. He regularly teaches on master's and diploma-level university courses. He has extensive experience teaching a wide variety of professionals including doctors, counsellors, nurses, probation officers, teachers and social workers.

Acknowledgements

We wish to thank a number of people for their support, encouragement and guidance in relation to this book. When the idea for this book emerged, we spoke to David B Cooper, who gave us tremendous support and practical advice on how to develop our idea into a book proposal. This help was invaluable and without it, this book may never have got off the ground. Once we contacted Radcliffe, Gillian Nineham and the rest of the Radcliffe team were consistently patient and helpful. They guided us through all the necessary stages and made a complicated process manageable – a feat for which we are truly grateful.

Additionally, we would like to thank the young people and their families whom we work with – through them we have learned so much. Various colleagues have provided support, ideas and feedback on various aspects of this project, which was so useful.

Individually, we would like to thank our spouses, families and friends for their support, encouragement and patience over the past 2 years.

Authors' note

When writing this book we sought to make a clear link to practice. A useful device for this is the use of case studies and vignettes in various chapters. In some cases we also have included sample dialogues between a worker and a young person. We would like to point out that these vignettes and quotes were made up by us to highlight a particular point or issue. In order to protect our clients' confidentiality we deliberately chose not to quote them or use their stories. However, based on our collective experience, we do believe that they are realistic vignettes which highlight the kind of problems our clients present with as well as typical comments they might say.

CHAPTER 1

Introduction

INTRODUCTION

Adolescent substance use is not a new phenomenon. It is routinely referenced in film and music. So common has it become that many people simply view it as a rite of passage – something every teen has to go through and come out the far side of. While this viewpoint is understandable in ways, it is important that we do not lose sight of the potentially disastrous effects that substance use can have for some teenagers. The repercussions can be drastic, including overdose, accidental injuries and criminal charges. For most teenagers who use substances, the negative effects tend to be less dramatic. Consequences such as poor school performance, early exit from education, dropping out of healthy activities such as sport and damage to family relationships are more usual. The effects of substance use will be discussed in more detail in the next chapter but, for now, consider the case example presented here.

Case example: Ivan's story

Ivan is a 17-year-old boy. Throughout his life his parents have not worried about him. He used to play football for the school and local club – while he was not the best player on his team he was pretty good. In the past, Ivan generally got on well in school and usually got at least Cs on his exams. He loves cars, motorbikes or pretty much anything with an engine. He has talked for a long time about becoming a mechanic once he leaves school. Overall, Ivan is a pretty unremarkable teenager – well liked, fairly popular and loved by his parents and siblings.

Two years ago, Ivan started drinking alcohol with friends most weekends, and more recently he began using cannabis. Twice, the police have detained him for being drunk, and he was arrested with a cannabis joint in his pocket 3 weeks ago. He is waiting to find out if he will be prosecuted for this or get another warning. He has not played football in months and his grades in school have suffered. Ivan has considered

---

dropping out of school, as he thinks he does not have the aptitude for it. He is skipping school regularly but he only has 6 months to graduation.

Ivan's parents are very worried about the changes they have seen in their son – they say he's not the boy they know and love. They have tried to talk with him about staying in school and to push him back into his hobbies and sports. These talks usually end in rows, as Ivan feels they do not listen to him. His parents are aware that he is drinking and smoking cannabis and have tried to discuss this with him. Ivan does not see it as a problem. Most of his friends smoke and drink about the same as him, 'so what's the big deal?' However, he concedes that none of his friends have been arrested before.

As we can see, Ivan's life is affected in a variety of ways. Many argue that the negative effects often attributed to drug misuse are not necessarily a result of the drug use. This may be true in some cases; however, as a general rule, those who use drugs are more likely to leave school early, get criminal charges, have mental health problems and have less satisfaction in life than those who do not use drugs. The more involved and heavy the drug use, the more likely the person is to experience these problems. Nonetheless, many teenagers use drugs or alcohol with few, if any, obvious negative effects. Consider Ivan's case and ask yourself the following:

- If Ivan continues on the current trajectory, what will his life be like in a year?
- Would a change in Ivan's drug use make a difference to him?

The obvious answers are that, while drugs may not have caused all of Ivan's problems, they are, at the very least, contributing to them. Life before drugs was healthier and happier than his current situation, and it is likely that things would improve somewhat if he stopped using. This book is designed to help those who work with adolescents and have concerns about substance use. The information contained herein should be as equally applicable to teenagers with severe drug or alcohol problems as to those with milder or experimental use.

SUBSTANCES OF ABUSE

Throughout the world, people take a plethora of substances to change how they feel. These mood-altering chemicals include tobacco, caffeine, alcohol, ecstasy, cannabis and heroin. Some products are legal (usually with age restrictions) and some are simply everyday substances that were never intended for use as a drug, such as sniffing glue. Throughout this book, we will use the word 'substances' to refer collectively to alcohol and drugs. Our definition of a substance is anything that is taken by someone for the purposes of changing his or her mood or perceptions. The drugs that teenagers use can be illegal (such as cocaine) or legal (such as diazepam), and even over-the-counter medications (such as codeine) are used to alter mood. Likewise, there are many ways in which drugs can be consumed, including eating, drinking, smoking and inhaling or sniffing. Chapter 3 provides an overview of the most commonly used substances of abuse.

It is important to note that this book is only focused on the misuse of mind-altering substances. We do not intend this book to focus on tobacco or caffeine, for the simple reason that it is exceptionally rare for a child to be referred to a substance abuse service for treatment of either tobacco or caffeine use. In recent years, there has been much discussion about the prevalence and consequences of a variety of other 'addictions', including the Internet, sex and gambling. Again, we have chosen not to explore these behavioural 'addictions' because of the rarity of referral.

A note on language

Throughout this book we use the term 'substance use' when discussing the use of substances in general. Other terms such as 'addiction' or 'substance abuse' are used when referring to use that is causing harm. When talking with adolescents about their substance use we advise caution. We are not keen on the use of terms such as 'addict' or 'alcoholic' because of the negative connotation attached to them. In our experience, clients rarely react well to being told they are an addict or that they are addicted. Even the phrase 'substance abuse' should be avoided. These terms can be perceived as judgemental by many and can lead to a defensive response that can be unhelpful. People do not like being labelled and frequently react with resistance to such comments. That being said, in many cases, people will readily admit that their drug or alcohol use is leading to, or at least contributing to, problems for them. Our recommendation is to avoid language that is likely to be perceived as judgemental. In comparison, discussing a substance that someone is using (as opposed to abusing) is less likely to cause problems. In doing this, we focus on a problem behaviour that can be, and is often, changed. Nevertheless, a working understanding of the variety of terms used is important for those who work with young people.

'Addiction' is one of the most commonly used terms and most people have a sense of its meaning. The problem is that it can mean different things to different people. In lay terms, people talk about being addicted to all sorts of things, including music, shopping, the gym, and so forth. In this way, addiction means finding it difficult to stop or cut down doing something, or simply spending a lot of time using this behaviour. To many people, addicts are seen as those with the most serious substance use problems – the intravenous drug user in Irvine Welsh's *Trainspotting*, the 'down-and-out' begging on the street. They often do not see someone who uses a drug once a week, even if it is causing that person problems, as being addicted. Addiction is also synonymous with withdrawal symptoms when the person stops taking the substance, like those experienced when someone withdraws from alcohol or heroin. Many young people see addiction in this chronic context and so do not see themselves as addicted. Perhaps they have never thought of their substance use as a problem and have never tried to stop. Likewise, cannabis, the most widely used illicit drug used by teens, does not have a dramatic withdrawal syndrome, leading many to assume it is not addictive.

Other terms also appear in the addiction-related literature and include 'substance misuse' and 'substance dependence'. The following is a quick description of these terms and how we understand them.

Substance use

A definition of substance use is inherent in the term. The person has used a substance. This may have been once or a hundred times. Many people, for example, use alcohol. This fact does not mean that it is causing them harm, or *not* causing them harm for that matter.

Substance misuse

Substance misuse is a common term used by professionals. Essentially, it goes a little further than substance use and states that the person is using the substance in an unhealthy way. For example, drinking alcohol to the point of getting hangovers or binge drinking could be described as misusing alcohol.

Substance abuse

Substance abuse is an official diagnosis for someone who is not only misusing the substance but also continuing to do so despite the fact it is causing significant harm to his or her life (e.g. debts or criminal charges). The World Health Organization uses the term 'harmful use' and this basically means the same thing.

Substance dependence

Substance dependence is another official diagnosis and is the most severe form of 'addiction' that can be diagnosed. Perhaps the main diagnostic difference between abuse and dependence is that there is often (but not always) evidence of tolerance (i.e. needing more of the drug to reach the same level of intoxication) and withdrawals upon stopping the drug where dependence is concerned. It is the presence of either withdrawals or tolerance that denotes whether someone is physically dependent. This is often referred to as being 'physically addicted'.

Lapse and relapse

When discussing substance use, relapse is often discussed, but in our experience it is important to separate a relapse from a lapse. Many people who stop using a substance have a slip. For example, someone who gives up cigarettes may smoke one or two at a party. While this is an unfortunate slip, this person has not reverted to his or her old pattern of use and so it could be termed a lapse. Should this person continue to smoke daily for days or weeks it could be termed a relapse.

As we can see, there is overlap in these terms and, in general, someone with dependence would be expected to be suffering more harm in more aspects of his or her life than someone with substance abuse. In practice, it can be very difficult to decide which diagnostic category an individual fits into, and it is not such an important issue. In the majority of cases, the level of substance use won't change the treatment dramatically, except in cases where severe withdrawal exists and requires medical intervention to help the person stop using a drug. Thankfully, such instances are not the norm with adolescents, but we have discussed medical interventions in greater depth in Chapter 10.

WHAT IS ADOLESCENCE?

When writing about adolescents, it is easy to use terms such as 'adolescence', 'teenagers' and 'young people' interchangeably. Arguably, this can lead to confusion because these terms are not always used in a consistent way. 'Teenagers' is a clear and simple term – it refers to the teenage years, ages 13–19. But what is a young person? Your answer to this question probably depends on your age. Some youth-centred health services work with individuals up until their mid-twenties. Adolescence is typically used to describe that period where a young person moves from being a child to being an autonomous adult. Most people probably see adolescence as being from about 12–19 years old. It could be argued that adolescence is moving further into the traditional adult years. In Western societies, greater proportions of the population are staying in education longer. A generation or so ago, most people left education at the end of second-level school, somewhere around the age of 17, and went out to work. As such, they were independent adults earning their own money. Now, more and more, people go on to further, third-level education with the result that they are dependent on their parents for longer – into their mid-twenties in some cases.

In this book, we have taken a pragmatic approach. We view adolescence as being the teenage years. The majority of the clients we see in our work fall between 15 and 18 years of age and so this book is aimed at this age group.

However, the information contained here should equally apply to all teens, and even some individuals outside this age range. For further discussion on adolescent development *see* Chapter 2.

IS ADOLESCENT DRUG USE DIFFERENT FROM ADULT DRUG USE?

The simple answer to this question is yes. We strongly believe that adolescents are not simply young adults. They are fundamentally different for a variety of reasons, and therefore they require an approach that is specifically aimed at them. When thinking about adolescent substance use bear in mind the following points.

- A person's brain development and emotional maturity is still developing throughout the teenage years and is not completed until the early twenties.
- The legal situation regarding drug use is different for teenagers (e.g. being unable to buy alcohol).
- Teenagers do not have the life experience to draw on that an adult has, making decision-making and problem-solving more difficult.
- Because they are minors, professionals owe teenagers a different duty of care. While it might be a legitimate decision to respect the autonomy of a 30-year-old and not interfere with their problematic drinking, it would not be okay to do so if they were 16.
- Adolescents rarely refer themselves for substance abuse treatment. Less than 3% of our referrals are self-referrals and, in most cases, the self-referrals we do get are returning clients rather than new clients.

As alluded to earlier, a debate continues in relation to teenagers and substance use. Many people argue that substance use as a teenager is simply part of growing up, a part of the developmental curve that is adolescence. This is often promoted in films where teenage drug and alcohol use are presented as the norm. Therefore, many do not see it as a major issue, as most teenagers grow out of it. Often, to illustrate this point, people will admit that they used drugs as a teen and that they turned out okay. This argument totally misses the point. It is the same as arguing that knowing one person who smoked cigarettes and lived to be 90 proves cigarettes are not bad for you. This is obviously nonsense and few people would make that argument. Just as everyone who smokes does not get cancer, not everyone who uses substances necessarily ends up with problems because of this substance use. Many *do* simply grow out of it. However, the earlier someone starts using, the more likely they are to have problems related to it. Many of you reading this book will be working with teenagers who have ended up in care, or emergency departments, coming to the attention of social services, doing poorly in school and so on. These teenagers are already suffering harm and have proven that they do not belong in the category of teens that use without any apparent consequences.

The other thing to bear in mind is that substance use among adolescents is not as common as some would claim. The European School Survey Project on Alcohol and Other Drugs (ESPAD) completes Europe-wide research on the activities of 15- and 16-year-olds. On average, across Europe 37% of 15- to 16-year-olds have been drunk in the past year and only 15% have been drunk more than once or twice! The same goes for cannabis – 13% have smoked cannabis in the past year and only 7% have used it more than once or twice.[1] These figures certainly refute the idea that everyone does it!

KEY POINTS

- Teenage drug use is associated with a variety of social, emotional, psychological and health risks. The earlier in life someone starts drug use, the greater these risks.
- It is not helpful to label a young person as addicted or alcoholic. This book will therefore use the term substance use.
- This book focuses on alcohol and drug use among teenagers.
- While adolescent substance use is relatively common, it is not the norm.
- Because drug use is associated with a variety of harms, it should be addressed whenever it becomes apparent that a teenager is using. Adopting a 'wait and see' approach is unlikely to be useful.

FURTHER READING

➡ *ESPAD Reports*: the ESPAD reports are completed across Europe with 15- and 16-year-olds. The same questions have been asked every 4 years since 1995 and so it is easy to see changes over time. Further information is available online (www.espad.org).

➡ *Health Behaviour in School-aged Children Reports*: this research project co-ordinated by the World Health Organization is similar to ESPAD in that it is a survey of teenagers in 43 countries every 4 years, most recently in 2009–10. It is carried out with 11-, 13- and 15-year-olds in each country and includes North America. The reports cover additional health-related topics like bullying, body image, diet and life satisfaction. There is a wealth of information online (www.hbsc.org).

REFERENCE

1 Hibell B, Guttormsson U, Ahlström S, *et al. The 2011 ESPAD Report: substance use among students in 36 European countries.* Stockholm: Swedish Council for Information on Alcohol and Other Drugs (CAN); 2012.

CHAPTER 2

Adolescence: a time of great change

Experimentation with substances typically commences during adolescence. In order to understand the phenomenon of substance use, it is therefore essential to have a good understanding of the teenage years.

CONSIDERING ADOLESCENTS AS APPRENTICE ADULTS

Adolescence is that much-maligned period of the lifespan that lies between childhood and adulthood. It is a time of dramatic change. The pace of development, both in terms of physical growth and in the acquisition of social skills, is probably only comparable with the rapid developments that occur during the first year of life.

As 10-year-old children we are entirely reliant on our parents to meet all of our basic needs. Our parents have great influence over our selection of peers and hobbies. By the time we reach 20, we are capable of managing a huge array of different social situations and challenges on our own. We have learned how to function independently in the complex world of adults. Therefore, the task as we journey through adolescence is to pick up the *skills* to equip ourselves for independent adult life.

People who are embarking on a period of skills acquisition are often called 'trainees' or 'apprentices'. These terms imply that a person is learning a range of additional skills to allow them to take on a new and independent role. We suggest that it is appropriate to conceptualise adolescents as *apprentice adults*.

Culture and adolescence

Notably, adolescence differs from culture to culture and, indeed, within cultures it changes over the decades.[1] Societies vary in the amount of time they allow young people to develop the skills to move towards independence. In affluent Western cultures, it can be argued that adolescence stretches into the early twenties as young people are given time to learn about themselves and the world before being required to take on the full burden of adult responsibilities. Many receive very substantial ongoing financial and other support from parents, permitting them to pursue higher education, for example.

In poorer cultures, young people are thrust into adult roles and responsibilities during their mid-teens because of financial imperatives such as the need to feed themselves and provide for their families. Also within Western cultures, at times of great difficulty and conflict, such as during wars, the years permitted for adolescence tends to be reduced, with young men in particular expected to take on huge responsibilities and obvious adult roles as soldiers at the age of 17 or 18.

Adolescence has always received bad press. About 400 years ago, in *The Winter's Tale*, William Shakespeare wished it away saying,

> I would there were no age between ten and three-and-twenty, or that youth would sleep out the rest; for there is nothing in the between but getting wenches with child, wronging the ancientry, stealing, fighting.[2]

In other words, Shakespeare wanted to put 10-year-olds into a coma and get them to emerge from it 13 years later as sensible adults, thereby bypassing the tumultuous intervening years.

Practice exercise: exploring adolescent stereotypes

We all have preconceived ideas about teenagers. Those beliefs are shaped by both our own experiences of teenagers and our culture's views of adolescence. Take a few moments to read the list of adjectives in Box 2.1 that can describe a person. Circle the five words that you think best characterise adolescents. Put another way, if an alien were to come to earth and ask you to describe typical adolescents, which five adjectives would you choose from this list?

BOX 2.1 Words used to describe adolescents

- Angry
- Cooperative
- Thoughtful
- Moody
- Considerate
- Energetic

- Defiant
- Independent
- Explosive
- Self-conscious
- Impulsive
- Reckless

- Secretive
- Hostile
- Helpful
- Argumentative
- Honest
- Rude

- Self-centred
- Demanding
- Empathic
- Pleasant
- Rebellious

- Unpredictable
- Polite
- Sex obsessed
- Ungrateful
- Confident

- Idealistic
- Creative
- Cautious

Having circled the five adjectives that you think best describe adolescence, now think of five teenagers you know. They may be your own children, cousins, nieces, nephews or neighbours' children. If you happen to work in a service that deals with troubled teenagers then avoid picking these, as they may not be typical teenagers. Reflect on these five real teenagers and consider their personalities and your interactions with them. Now return to the same list of adjectives in Box 2.1 and underline the five adjectives that *best* describe the characteristics of the specific teenagers you have thought of.

We have conducted this exercise numerous times with adults and have found that there is a marked tendency to circle many of the negative adjectives to describe the typical teenager. The most frequently endorsed items are 'moody', 'self-conscious' and 'rebellious'. In fact, we have found that 80% of the adjectives selected are negative. However, in the second part of the exercise, when people are encouraged to think about real teenagers known to them in their day-to-day lives, they end up endorsing mainly the positive adjectives. The three most commonly chosen words are 'pleasant', 'helpful' and 'thoughtful' and positive adjectives account for 75% of the selected words.

What this exercise demonstrates is that we tend to have a negative stereotypical view of adolescents. It is unfortunate for teenagers that they live in a world of adults who view them so poorly, despite their generally pleasant, helpful and thoughtful behaviour. This dim view of adolescents is not unique to the twenty-first-century world. A famous social commentator wrote the following description of teenagers:

> The children now love luxury; they have bad manners, contempt for authority . . . disrespect for elders . . . they contradict their parents . . . and terrorise their teachers.

While many read this and think it applies to the contemporary world, it was in fact written by Socrates over 2000 years ago. Society has grappled with the challenges posed by teenagers throughout the millennia.

Comic depictions of teenagers

We, as ordinary members of society, are not the only groups who negatively stereotype teenagers. Perpetuating these stereotypes, many of our favourite comedians make a good living from lampooning teenage behaviours. Think of Harry Enfield's huffing Kevin, and Matt Lucas' anarchic Vicky Pollard of *Little Britain* fame. They present loud, demanding, self-centred, precocious, angry and impatient characterisations of the teenage years. These are features that we *do* occasionally encounter in *some* teenagers. Perhaps we also recall being a bit this way ourselves. However, because these caricatures are so extreme, they probably contribute to our excessively negative view of a typical teenager.

Development is not simply a passive process

Like all phases of life, adolescent development is not simply a passive process. Individuals do not *automatically* pick up the same range of skills and competencies at the same pace as they move through their teenage years.

Bright, socially competent children are likely to develop further skills of independent functioning more rapidly than their less clever and less socially skilled peers. They are likely to be selected by their peers to be leaders and they will also be chosen by adults to act, for example, as prefects and leaders within school and club settings. This then gives them quite a different experience than their less socially skilled non-prefect peers. As they are given the opportunity to experience leadership roles, this further develops their already superior social and organisational skills. Essentially, a teenager's own intrinsic competencies will influence the opportunities that he or she is afforded during adolescence. From these new and novel challenges, additional skills will be obtained.

Obviously, at the other extreme, less socially competent teenagers, who are perhaps prone to anger and who struggle with peer relationships, may find themselves marginalised within their peer group. If combined with a lack of academic ability and educational expectation, this is likely to result in a poor experience of school. Such teenagers can get into repeated conflict with teachers and are therefore more likely to drift out of school. Their departure from the school environment does not mean that they will fail to pick up any social skills during their teenage years. Nonetheless, the skills they acquire are often learned from older, more delinquent peers and may involve them engaging in increasing antisocial behaviour in order to gain status among their peer group. This, in turn, brings them into conflict with 'mainstream' society and often draws the attention of the criminal justice system. The story of Kevin and Tim in Box 2.2 highlights some of these points, albeit for two quite ordinary teenagers.

BOX 2.2 Kevin and Tim: a journey into adolescence

Kevin and Tim are lifelong friends who live on the same road. They are 13 and have just moved from the local primary school into the first year in secondary school. Kevin is a talented soccer player and gets on well with his classmates, both boys and girls. He finds school work fairly easy and is an average pupil. Tim is tall and quieter than Kevin. He likes computer games and is very good at maths. He likes playing soccer and tennis, although he has never been great at either. He has become more physically awkward since he had a recent growth spurt. He has a good group of male friends, whom he has known for years, but he is a bit somewhat shy when meeting new people. Although he fancies Jennifer, who lives nearby, he gets self-conscious around her.

Kevin becomes captain of the under-14 school soccer team. His dad is very proud of his soccer achievements. He is well known and well liked by the older boys at school. He does his homework most of the time, and he doesn't cause any problem in class. His grades slip slightly. Tim studies quite hard. He continues to do well at maths and really likes science. He tried out for the soccer team but dropped out of training after he spent a couple of matches on the sideline for the 'B' team. He still plays some tennis in the local club and kicks a ball around with his friends when they are hanging out in the park. He still gets on well with Kevin, but he makes excuses not to join him at the monthly teenage disco. Tim still only has eyes for Jennifer, but she doesn't seem interested in him. Kevin goes to the discos and has begun dating a girl from another school, although he's not taking it too seriously.

Kevin and Tim are both entirely normal teenagers. Each will arrive into adulthood with the necessary skills to manage independent life, although their areas of strength may differ. Partly because of their different areas of natural talent, their journey through adolescence will differ and the pace at which they pick up the skills that equip them for independent life will vary. Their friendship is likely to endure.

Kevin is fortunate to have above-average soccer and social skills. As he has these skills he is then given opportunities to develop them further. Tim is not so lucky. His soccer and social skills are below average. People often opt out of things they are not so good at. Tim quits the soccer team and is inclined to opt out of some social situations and is not given the opportunity to tackle others. As a result, the gap between Tim and Kevin, in terms of both soccer ability and social skills, widens further. Those with intrinsic talents are given further opportunities to develop these natural skills. People with intrinsic deficiencies may withdraw or be removed from opportunities to develop skills in those areas.

Developmental psychologists call this phenomenon 'a transactional process in temporal progress'. It is not unique to adolescence and can be seen throughout the lifespan. For example, infants smile automatically at anything that resembles a human face from the age of about 6 weeks. Most adults like smiley children. That being said, children differ in their tendency to smile and the children who are most smiley tend to get more adult attention. It is through engaging adults in this way that children receive nurturing, listen to language and engage in play. This interaction has a positive influence on their motor development, and through listening to adults talking it provides them with an opportunity to learn language and communication. Hence, the smiley baby has an advantage over his or her less-smiley counterpart.

THE TEENAGE BRAIN IS A WORK IN PROGRESS

In the past decade, science has shed new light on adolescent development. Recent research has demonstrated that the adolescent brain continues to develop throughout the teenage years.[3] In fact, these changes to the adolescent brain are perhaps essential in developing the more sophisticated thinking skills demonstrated by older teenagers. It is now clear that during the teenage years the brain cells, or neurons, establish new and more elaborate connections between one another.[4] These new connections between neurons are maintained if they are being utilised by the person, and connections that are not utilised are gradually pruned away to make the brain a more finely tuned and efficient entity.

Deterioration in some skills around puberty

Parents sometimes lament the changes that they see in their teenage children. Some parents describe a dramatic change in their child who was previously chatty, interactive and pleasant. They describe their teenager becoming distant, with communication almost confined to grunting. While such observations are probably exaggerated, the brain research does give some clues as to what may be happening.

During adolescence, as the brain develops it can become temporarily less efficient.[4] This temporary decline in functioning has been demonstrated by research. For example, an adolescent's ability to quickly recognise facial emotions (such as 'happy', 'confused', 'frightened' and 'shocked') actually deteriorates in the early teenage years. This deterioration corresponds with this period of brain development during puberty where new connections are made and some pruned. Performance on this task later improves and increases to a level that exceeds that demonstrated in childhood. Put simply, the brain gets worse before it gets better.

The brain doesn't fully mature until the early twenties

This process of development occurs within the brain over the teenage years, progressing from the back and bottom towards the upper parts of the frontal lobes. The frontal lobes represent that portion of the brain that is involved in complex thinking skills. These include the skills that allow us to interact, communicate and problem-solve in the sophisticated way we do as adults. The frontal lobes do not appear to fully mature until the early twenties.

This process of brain change during adolescence is hugely important. It seems to explain the improvement in thinking ability that developmental psychologists, such as Piaget, first described 40 years ago.[5] It may also explain why substance use by teenagers seems to be much more harmful than similar levels of drug or alcohol use by people in their late twenties.

The fact that the brain matures in an uneven manner, with frontal lobes being last to fully develop, is important and goes some way to explain some features of the adolescent years.[6] Parts of the limbic system mature much earlier than the frontal lobes. The limbic system is important in driving human behaviour. It is like the engine in a car. The frontal lobes have the job of screening impulsive desires and weighing up the pros and cons of behaviour options. The frontal lobes are like the brakes in a car. Children have less well-developed limbic systems and frontal lobes but importantly, the 'engine' and the 'brakes' are in balance. Adults have well-developed and powerful limbic systems and frontal lobes. In other words, the powerful 'engine' is counterbalanced with a strong 'braking system', just as supercars tend to have massive brake discs. In adolescents, the limbic system (engine) becomes powerful before the frontal lobe (braking system) has fully developed. If a car were manufactured with the engine of a Ferrari but the brakes of a Ford Escort, it would be hard to drive. While it might cope okay with straight motorways in light traffic, it would be difficult to handle and liable to crash on poorer roads and in heavier traffic.

Therefore, nature has designed teenagers to go, and not to stop. While this may seem cruel, it does make sense in that they are required, by nature, to take on new challenges and to be less aware of risks. Where does the adolescent albatross get the courage to leap from the nest high on the cliff that first time when it has never flown before? While the challenges faced by human adolescents are not so stark, they need a little bit of nerve to go into town on their own that first time, to ask a girl out for the first time, and so on.

While nature has designed the human brain to have this mismatch between its engine and braking system, there is going to be substantial individual

difference. Some teenagers may experience early maturation of the limbic system (engine) and delayed maturation of the frontal lobes (braking system).
These teenagers, therefore, have a wide and prolonged mismatch between
the engine and the brakes, and will likely demonstrate substantial risk-taking
behaviour. In other teenagers, there may be little gap between the maturation
of these two brain areas, thereby reducing the likelihood of risky behaviour.
While science is just beginning to shed light on the neurobiological processes
that underpin risky and impulsive behaviour, we are decades away from having any biological 'treatment' or intervention for young people who have a big
mismatch between their limbic system and frontal lobes.

Apart from the brain, the other and more obvious physical change over adolescence is puberty. This is the process whereby boys and girls mature sexually,
and thereby develop the capacity to procreate. *See* Box 2.3 for a more detailed
discussion on puberty.

BOX 2.3 Puberty

Puberty is the process of development of secondary sexual characteristics and it
is a key feature of adolescence. Both genders grow rapidly during puberty. The
rate of growth in height and weight during puberty is second only to that seen in
infancy. In both genders there is growth of pubic and axillary hair. In girls, breasts
develop and the menstrual cycle commences. In boys, the voice becomes deeper,
the testes and penis grow in size and sperm production commences.

The period of most obvious physical change lasts about 4 years in both
genders. Puberty starts on average 2 years earlier in girls. It normally occurs
during the age range of 8–18 years in girls and 9–19 years in boys.

The hormonal systems are present from birth but they remain suppressed
during childhood. The key female hormones are oestrogen and progesterone.
The key male hormone is testosterone. There is a slow detectable rise in these
hormones starting at age 5–8 years of age. Puberty appears to be 'switched
on' once a person achieves a critical metabolic level.[1] Factors influencing this
metabolic level include the fat–muscle ratio and body weight.

Girls have been starting menstruation progressively earlier for over a century
until the 1970s in Western countries, as nutrition improved. Data from the
nineteenth century suggests that undernourished boys and girls finished their
growth 4–5 years later and ended up shorter in stature than their well-nourished
contemporaries. Both final height and pubertal onset appear now to have levelled
off, suggesting that the current nutrition/health is optimal. The limiting factor on
age of onset of puberty across teenagers is now primarily genetic.

Are there psychosocial influences on puberty?
Some research suggests that adolescents may respond to family discord by maturing quickly, leaving the 'unhappy situation' earlier, to find other relationships outside the home. Animal research has found that continued close association with a parent delays maturation, while forceful removal leads to earlier onset of puberty.

Influence of timing of puberty
American research indicates that early-maturing boys and late-maturing girls do best academically. Early-maturing girls are 'more popular' with boys. Early-maturing girls tend to be less satisfied with bodies in later adolescence, as they tend to be shorter.

THE VITAL ROLE OF SCHOOL IN ADOLESCENT DEVELOPMENT

School provides a crucial role in adolescent development. Most people view the primary function of school as the provision of education. In our view, the most important function of school is the provision of a contained, structured environment in which children can hone and gradually improve their broadening repertoire of social skills beyond the safety of the family home.

The transition into the 'chaos' of senior or secondary school

While education structures differ from country to country, there is usually a division between junior and senior schools. In general, progression to senior school occurs around the onset of adolescence, at 11–13 years. Adolescents face significant challenges in this transition and a minority of young people struggle. In junior school the student's day is regimented. The child has the same teacher all day, typically the teacher will go through the same routine each day, and the child will sit in the same seat and will be surrounded by the same peers. Life is predictable.

This routine changes in senior school, as teenagers have to negotiate a subject timetable that varies daily. Each subject may require a move to a different classroom. They have a multitude of teachers, each of whom inevitably has a different teaching style and approach to discipline. They sit in a different location in each class and are surrounded by different peers. Learning a number of new subjects is another challenge. They move from a position of being the oldest in the school to being the 'babies' once again.

In many ways it is remarkable that the majority of teenagers meet this challenge without significant difficulty. However, a significant minority fall by the wayside. Some teenagers become so overwhelmed that they start refusing to go to school, preferring instead the safety, familiarity and predictability of home.[7] It is for these reasons that school refusal can spike again around the age of 13. Other teenagers become disillusioned with school and end up in conflict with one or more of their teachers. This can result in them leaving school, despite the fact that they may have had quite a reasonable record in junior school.

Schools fostering a growing independence in teenagers

As teenagers progress through the senior school system they find that they are given increased autonomy and freedom in a phased way. They are given additional privileges and independence to match the development of their social competence. They are encouraged to become more involved in the school community and activities. Many are supported in taking a leadership role in looking after younger students. The best schools provide an environment in which teenagers can explore a range of sporting or social activities. This gives all pupils the opportunity to discover their talents and to find areas that stimulate, challenge and interest them. It also provides opportunities to meet like-minded peers and establish a broad range of friendships.

School also requires them to be surrounded by peers who may have different values, beliefs and behaviours. They are not going to like everybody and not everyone is going to like them. While this clearly poses a challenge, it also gives them the opportunity to develop the skills to survive and manage relationships with others with whom they have little in common.

PROGRESSIVE INCREASE IN CONFIDENCE AND COMPETENCE

It is useful to think about the relationship between teenagers' growing competence and their escalating confidence. During normal adolescent development teenagers pick up an increasing range of social skills. These enhanced social competencies allow them to interact with authority, peers, family and their community in a more sophisticated manner. With this growing competence there is likely to be an associated increase in confidence in their ability to take on these and future challenges. Consequently confidence and competence generally increase in parallel throughout adolescence.

As with any apprentice, it is important that those who provide the mentoring continually assess competence and confidence. Where both are progressing at a decent rate and in parallel, mentoring is easy. Unfortunately, some apprentices are poor judges of their competence and may overestimate it, because of excessive confidence. An apprentice plumber with an inflated sense of his or her own ability may take on jobs that he or she is not equipped to manage alone. An overly confident apprentice doctor may start diagnosing serious ill-nesses and initiating complex treatments without checking adequately with his or her supervisor. While such apprentices may make the right decision *most* of the time, they are still prone to error. Where problems arise because of their poor previous decisions, they lack the ability to recognise and manage these, and things can get very messy. At the other end of the spectrum, sometimes an apprentice will demonstrate a level of confidence that is too low for his or her level of competence. This can result in reluctance in taking on new challenges and constantly checking with his or her supervisor. While not dangerous, this type of apprentice inevitably progresses more slowly and requires a different style of mentoring.

Confidence–competence mismatch and its problems

Overly confident teenagers, who are fearless and willing to take on any new challenge, may find themselves in situations that are really out of their depth. For example, a 13-year-old girl who goes to a disco for 16-year-olds may strug-gle to manage the advances of older boys. Many, if not most, teenagers will occasionally put themselves in situations that are a bit out of their depth. Indeed, most of us will look back on these situations as useful learning expe-riences. However, if a teenager constantly puts him- or herself into situations that are beyond his or her competence, the teenager is likely to run out of luck at some point. Some adults rationalise this persistent risk-taking behaviour as an opportunity to learn from mistakes. Nonetheless, the consequences of their poor choices can have serious and long-term consequences. In general, we don't employ the strategy of getting apprentices to learn from their mistakes as a cen-tral part of their training. Just as an overly confident apprentice plumber will need closer monitoring, so too does the overly confident teenager.

A confidence–competence mismatch in the opposite direction is also problematic with our apprentice adults. Overly cautious teenagers, who lack confidence to take on new social challenges, miss out on the social learn-ing opportunities that come with this broader array of social interactions. Consequently, by the time they arrive into adulthood they are less capable of managing the full repertoire of adult social situations than their more confi-dent peers.

FRIENDSHIPS DURING THE TEENAGE YEARS

Friends are important and can change considerably during the adolescent years. Typically, in early childhood, friendships are determined by shared interest in activities. During adolescence, friendships tend to become more sophisticated and we choose our friends based upon shared values and 'feeling understood' by them. The importance of establishing an emotional connection and some sense of empathy with one's friends becomes increasingly important in maintaining friendships.

Emotional literacy and empathy

During the teenage years people become better able to label their own emotional state. Generally, a 6-year-old describes his mood as simply being good or bad. However, during adolescence we become better at discriminating between different emotions, recognising the difference between shame, anxiety, sadness and anger. Just as we grow in our ability to label our own emotions, we also increase in our ability to recognise and predict the emotional responses of others.[4] This capacity to label our own emotions and empathise with others constitutes important skills that permit us to develop the more sophisticated friendships of older adolescence.

Teenagers who don't understand or who struggle to empathise with their peers will be less able to develop close peer relationships. Unfortunately, this problem tends to become self-perpetuating. Their failure to establish close friendships denies them the experience of such meaningful relationships, preventing them from learning how to develop and sustain future friendships.

Identity formation: 'Who am I?'

Typically, 7-year-old boys follow the same football team and want to have the same career as their dad. They will tend to have similar values and opinions to their parents. As teenagers they begin to attach increasing weight to the values, beliefs and views of their peers. This may involve completely discarding, albeit on a temporary basis, their parents' values. It is often through peers that they will begin to explore their own identity and to find the values, beliefs and behaviours that fit for them. In the company of peers, they encounter different ways of dressing and different music styles. Their circle of friends may change as part of this process of exploration as the teenager begins to figure out how they see themself and how they want the world to see them. While it is something we may choose to forget as adults, we all engaged in this exploration to some extent, even those of us who were cautious by disposition. You may recall some fashion faux pas from your own adolescence. The practice exercise in Box 2.4 may help to remind you. One big advantage we have as adults in our work with teenagers is that we were once in their shoes. However, as adults we often forget what was really going on for us at that time. Rewinding the clock a few decades may help you to understand teenagers a little better.

BOX 2.4 Exploring our identity as adolescents

Take a moment to think back on your own journey through adolescence or, if possible, discuss it with another adult. Recall a time when you decided to make a change. It might have been your hairstyle, your clothes or telling your friends about a music album you had bought. Perhaps you decided to take up a new hobby or activity, or to break into a different group of friends. In retrospect it might seem quite trivial, but at the time it probably felt like a big deal.

- Think or talk about what influenced you to make the change in the first place. Was it friends, family, parents, television or someone 'famous'?
- What, or who, were you worried about in advance?
- How did it work out?
  - What was the actual reaction from your friends, parents, and so forth?
  - Did you continue or did you stop, and who or what influenced your decision?

Peer pressure: both good *and* bad

Peer pressure gets a great deal of coverage in the press and is a subject of substantial discussion anytime teenagers are talked about. Because teenagers value the views and opinions of their peers, they are likely to engage in behaviours that are endorsed and approved of by their friends. We should also remember that this is not confined to adolescence. As adults, we too attach weight to the views and opinions of others.

Oftentimes we view peer pressure negatively. The term 'peer influence' is probably better, as it's certainly not always a negative influence. It can be very healthy. It simply depends on the peer group with whom the teenager happens to affiliate.

If the teenager hangs around with a rule-breaking, drug-using peer group, he or she is likely to be drawn into behaviours that are socially deviant. This can have a potentially destructive influence on his or her development. Yet a teenager, who may have some precocious or adventurous tendencies, may affiliate with a group of more cautious, sensible and responsible teenagers. These peers are likely to disapprove and to criticise the teenager any time he or she exhibits any of the dangerous or antisocial behaviour to which he or she is prone. In such instances, the peer influence or peer pressure can certainly be positive.

IMPLICATIONS OF VARIATIONS IN PACE OF DEVELOPMENT

As with all apprentices, there is variability in the pace at which individual apprentice adults acquire the skills to equip themselves for independent adult functioning. As a society we are most aware of these developmental differences in early childhood when children are learning to walk and talk. Most infants typically have their first words at around 12–14 months. On the other hand, many children do not begin to speak until they are 2 years old. Similarly, while children typically begin taking their first steps around the age of 1 year, some walk at 10 months while others don't take any steps until they are 2 years old. We don't blame children for this variation in pace, we simply recognise it as a difference. Children who do not begin to walk or talk until they are 21–24 months old are not viewed as lazy or stupid. We accept a natural amount of variability in development.

Variability in athletic skills is accepted

Teachers and parents are quick to recognise that older children and teenagers vary in their athletic skills. There are some children who will make the basketball team without any great effort. There are others who remain mediocre players despite putting in huge efforts at training. We don't condemn them for their modest performance, especially if we see them trying so hard. We just view them as different. Generally, we continue to give them the opportunity to improve as a player by getting them to play on the 'B' or 'C' team.

Teenagers with 'naturally' poor social skills are blamed for them

Both natural talent and practice influence performance on the pitch, but no amount of the latter can compensate for a major deficiency in the former. It is the same for social skills. However, aloof socially awkward teenagers are often viewed as having *chosen* to behave this way.

Children vary significantly in the pace at which they master emotional regulation. Following minor disappointments, some teenagers can react with intense anger or sadness, while most will simply shrug their shoulders and move on. They also differ in their ability to empathise with others. This can result in some being seen as lazy, deliberately moody, callous, cruel or insensitive to their family and peers. Their socially gauche or difficult behaviour is seen as a choice. This is unfortunate because it means that the underlying deficit is missed.

If the underlying deficit were detected, the ideal response from school, family and community would be to support the teenager by providing them with opportunities to acquire the skills they are deficient in. Instead, they may be rejected and become socially isolated, or else they affiliate with other angry youngsters. Both outcomes tend to become self-perpetuating.

WHY TEENAGERS DO RECKLESS THINGS

Having stated earlier that teenagers get a bad press and tend to be stereotyped negatively, it is still a reality that adolescents do make poorer choices more often than adults. They are more likely to engage in risky behaviours and cause harm to themselves or others as a result. While we have a propensity to blame teenagers for making these choices and engaging in behaviours that appear reckless, there are in fact logical explanations as to why they mess up more frequently than adults.

1 Concrete thinking

As outlined earlier, teenagers' brains have not developed completely. In childhood and early teenage years there is a leaning towards 'concrete thinking', as described by the developmental psychologist Piaget.[5] This style of thinking is characterised as seeing the world in black and white. Behaviour is viewed as good or bad. There is difficulty in taking mitigating factors into account. For example, stealing a big cake is seen as worse than stealing a small bun, even if the former is taken to feed a starving family and the latter is robbed just to throw at a friend.

During adolescence as the frontal lobes mature and develop, there is the development of what Piaget calls 'formal operational thinking'. This improved cognitive style means the adolescents can think more latterly. There is an ability to extrapolate from past events and apply that knowledge to current challenges. An improved ability to predict the consequences of current behaviours based on experiences of similar situations also emerges. There is a greater ability to understand and anticipate the motives behind our own and others' behaviour.

Formal operational thinking is established by the mid-teenage years but, as always, there is variability from person to person. Teenagers who have not yet developed this more mature style of thinking are more likely to make poor choices when presented with challenging situations or difficulties in interpersonal relationships. There is a particular inclination for teenagers to make poor choices as they head into difficult or risky situations. These poor choices can, to some extent, 'dig themselves further into a hole'.

2 Avoidance

The stereotypical coping response of early adolescence is avoidance.[1] This may manifest itself as going to one's room, slamming the door shut, and turning music on loudly following a row with a teacher, parent, friend or girlfriend. The problem is ignored and the teenagers just wait for it to go away. This head-in-the-sand, ostrich response is not nearly as effective as the more proactive coping strategies that most of us have developed as adults.

3 Omnipotence: being blind to danger

Although omnipotence is a characteristic that can be seen throughout an individual's life, it is typically associated with adolescence. Elkind[8] described it in the 1960s. Individuals who demonstrate omnipotence display invulnerability to the adverse consequences of risk behaviour. While they may be aware that there is some inherent risk in the behaviour they are engaging in, they overestimate their own competence to manage these situations. It is an example of the competence–confidence mismatch discussed earlier, where confidence is well in excess of competence.

A sense of omnipotence is probably the main explanation for increased road deaths among young men aged between 17 and 21 years. When they get behind the wheel, although they might well be aware that there are risks in driving too fast, they overestimate their own driving ability. Consequently, they are inclined to drive too fast for the circumstances and, on occasion, crash, killing or injuring themselves and/or others in the process. The brain development research in recent decades has demonstrated that the brain's engine matures before its braking system. This provides a possible biological explanation for the confidence–competence mismatch.[6]

4 The value of life experience

> It is a pity that, as one gradually gains experience, one loses one's youth.
>
> —*Vincent van Gogh (1853–90)*

By the time adults reach their mid-thirties, they have about 15 years of really useful life experience under their belts, having had a reasonable amount of autonomy since their late teens. During those years they have been presented with a wide range of social challenges and situations. They have hopefully learned a lot along the way about how society works and how relationships operate. Consequently, for any novel situation they find themselves in, or new challenge they encounter, adults are likely to have been in a similar situation previously. They can draw upon this wealth of experience to guide them in managing and dealing with the current dilemma.

If they are presented with a problem that is particularly complex, they can turn to their peers for advice on possible courses of action. Their friends are likely to be of a similar age and, as a result, they can draw upon their few decades of life experience when dispensing advice to their adult friend.

It is very different for a young teenager who may well be encountering a conflict with authority or a difficulty in a loving relationship for the first time. Such events can become overwhelming in large part because the teenager has little past experience to draw upon in meeting these challenges. Accordingly, the teenager will draw upon other knowledge or learning. This may well be based upon what he or she has seen on television soaps such as *Home and Away*, *EastEnders* or *The Hills*. When the teenager turns to others for advice it is likely to be peers, as indeed it is for adults. However, unlike adults, their friends are young teens who are equally inexperienced in managing life's difficulties. Hence, the advice these friends dispense may not be great. Thus, teenagers will mess up and make poor choices much more frequently than we do as adults.

BOX 2.5 *Romeo and Juliet*: a teenage love story

Romeo and Juliet, probably the most famous love story, is actually about teenage love. Juliet is 13 years old, and although Romeo's exact age is not stated it is implied that he is about 16. Juliet, experiencing intense emotional attraction for the first time becomes rapidly overwhelmed by it. Romeo, although bemoaning the failure of Rosaline to return his affections at the start of the play, quickly forgets her once he meets the beautiful Juliet. He is overtaken by an all-powerful desire for Juliet once he knows that she reciprocates his love. Within a day they decide that they must be together forever and they plan to marry. There are obstacles in their path and they hatch a convoluted plan to negotiate these. As neither can bear the prospect of being without the other, they take quite extreme risks to be together, and when they ultimately believe this to be no longer possible, death becomes an attractive option.

Romeo and Juliet did not *know* from personal experience how to manage strong feelings of love. They did not *know* from their own experience how to resolve complex interpersonal problems. They may have been advised by adults about these things. However, neither of them had ever before negotiated the challenges that they faced. Hence they made some reckless choices and their story ended tragically.

5 The stress and hazards of being surrounded by other teenagers

An additional challenge of being a teenager is the fact that other teenagers normally surround you. To highlight what we mean, let's use the analogy of skiing. As one gains competence in skiing one is less likely to fall over and will manage steeper slopes. The skier begins to handle bumps and undulations in the ground without overreacting or losing balance. Similarly, if another skier has fallen, the first skier can carefully and easily negotiate his or her way around the faller without injuring him- or herself or the other skier. As the skier becomes even more competent and confident, he or she can do much more than just avoid colliding with the fallen skier. The skier can stop and offer assistance by bringing skis and poles to the fallen skier. This contrasts greatly with the chaos on the nursery slopes. On the nursery slopes you are there because you are a beginner, lacking the basic skills. Unfortunately, equally incompetent skiers surround you. Consequently, it is in this environment that accidents and collisions are most likely to occur. If someone falls in front of you as he or she struggles to learn the basics too, there is a tendency to roll over and collapse yourself or else to just plough into the other skier, hurting both the other skier and yourself. While the desire might be there, there is certainly little or no ability to assist the fallen skier.

The start of secondary school is very similar to the nursery slope. Both in and out of school, these young students are surrounded by other teenagers who are also grappling with and trying to manage the increased independence and freedom that they are gaining. They are all at the beginning of their adulthood apprenticeships. While some will be more capable than others, they are all at the very early stages of developing competence in terms of interacting with peers, building mature relationships, consolidating their sense of themselves as individuals and dealing with authority. Ultimately, each individual teenager is surrounded by others who are inclined to mess up, make mistakes, be socially gauche and perhaps socially cruel. These scenarios are not unlike the skiers falling around you. Similarly, where one's peers are beginning to struggle or to hit difficulty, the inexperienced 14-year-old classmate has problems avoiding getting embroiled in the conflict. Compared with adults and older teenagers, the 14-year-old is less able to anticipate the difficulties that his or her peers may be heading towards and so less capable of assisting them when they do hit problems. Although challenging, just as there is no real choice in avoiding the nursery slope if one wants to learn to ski, teenagers have no choice but to endure this somewhat awkward and stressful phase of the lifespan.

As with any apprenticeship, it is always helpful to get off to a good start. It is important that parents, teachers and others mentoring these apprentice adults quickly spot the struggling teenagers. Those teenagers will need additional mentoring and monitoring to support them in catching up with their peers.

DESPITE THE CHALLENGES, 'TURMOIL' IS NOT THE NORM

Despite the teenage stereotypes, the caricatures by comedians, and the writings of Shakespeare, Socrates and more recent social commentators, it is important to remember that *turmoil and great difficulty is not the norm during the teenage years*. There was a view that adolescence is an inevitably difficult and tumultuous time. Research in recent decades reveals that this is not the case in most circumstances. It is probably no more than 25%–30% of teenagers who encounter substantial emotional or behavioural difficulty during the teenage years.[1] Put another way, 70%–75% have a relatively uncomplicated journey through adolescence.

There are reasons to be concerned about the stereotypical view that adolescence is always a dreadfully difficult time. Real difficulties that are occurring for a teenager are more likely to be dismissed and ignored than at any other stage of the lifespan.[9] When teenagers, or their parents, turn to others to seek assistance in managing intense emotional upset or behavioural difficulty, there is a risk that relatives, friends and some health professionals may offer inappropriate reassurance that it is 'just the teenage phase'. As a consequence, problems that would not be ignored in an 8-, 28- or 88-year-old are often allowed to persist for longer and may become more entrenched by the time assistance is sought.

PARENTING OF TEENAGERS

Psychologists have described four main styles of parenting, based upon Baumrind's[10] two orthogonal dimensions. These dimensions are *responsiveness* and *demandingness*. Responsiveness indicates the sensitivity of the parent to the child and priority given to warmth in the relationship. Demandingness indicates the presence of high expectations regarding behaviour and active efforts to ensure appropriate behaviour by the child. Based upon their position on these two dimensions, parents can be categorised into one of four different categories (*see* Figure 2.1). These are Authoritarian, Authoritative, Laissez-faire and Neglectful.[11] There are questionnaires that assess parenting style, such as the Parental Authority Questionnaire.[12] There is general agreement that authoritative parenting constitutes the best parenting style for most children and adolescents.

Adolescence is not simply a time of challenge and change for the teenager. It is also a time of transition for parents. The parenting approach that is effective and appropriate for an 8-year-old may not work well with a 16-year-old.

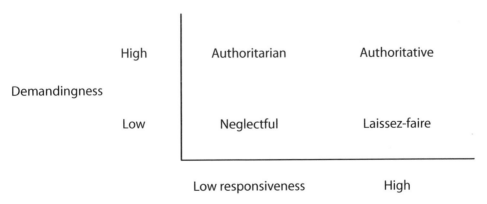

FIGURE 2.1 Baumrind's categorisation of parenting styles

Even parents who adhere to the authoritative style need to make subtle shifts within this approach, especially along the demandingness dimension. With 8-year-olds it is generally appropriate for parents to use a style that involves the parent laying down clear rules that are not open to negotiation. The parent determines what is acceptable and unacceptable. The parent decides how desired behaviour will be rewarded and what sanctions will be imposed for breaches of rules. However, it is inappropriate to use the harsh punishments that can be associated with authoritarian parenting.

Ideally, during adolescence parents alter their approach slightly to reflect the growing abilities and independence of their son or daughter. Nevertheless, the parent remains clearly in charge, establishing the parameters beyond which behaviours cannot proceed. However, within these boundaries there is increasing room for negotiation. The amount of negotiation and discussion should gradually increase as the teenager grows in competence. Parental responsiveness to their child's needs should be prominent throughout both childhood and adolescence.

Dangers of being too authoritarian

Parents often have children of varying age. Therefore they are required to move seamlessly and effortlessly from a more dogmatic approach when dealing with the issues relating to an 8-year-old to the more negotiated approaches required for a 16-year-old.[11] Some parents don't demonstrate this flexibility and this can pose problems. Conflict in the parent–child relationship is a common reason for referral to child and adolescent mental health services. Occasionally during our careers in adolescent mental health, we have met families where the main problem seemed to originate in the parents' inability to move away from an authoritarian parenting style. Given that teenagers are required to make steps towards independence during their adolescence, while also exploring their identity through engaging in new behaviours, this inevitably brings conflict.

Laissez-faire parenting and its pitfalls

It is important that parents do not move too far towards a laissez-faire parenting approach. This approach is particularly inappropriate for teenagers who are precocious and adventurous. Laissez-faire parents place great value in being warm and affectionate with their children (high responsiveness), while handing over a huge amount of responsibility for behaviour to the child (low demandingness). There is minimal monitoring, few rules and few consequences, believing the child will learn from his or her own mistakes. The parent responds to these mistakes with much compassion but no new restrictions. It may work well with teenagers who are mature, competent and strongly inclined towards positive social behaviours.

There is substantial intrinsic difference between teenagers in terms of their personality, learning style and propensity to take risks. Such differences can manifest within siblings in the one family. A parenting style that may have worked fine with older children (e.g. laissez-faire) may not work for later children because of these intrinsic differences between children. Parents need to *adapt their parenting style to the specific teenager* in front of them.

A laissez-faire approach clearly can cause problems where freedoms and independence are given that are beyond children's ability to manage. They *attain autonomy beyond their competence.* This can lead to a vicious cycle of escalating difficulties, leading to a range of emotional and behavioural difficulties, and increasing risk behaviour. By the time parents spot the hazards it can be extremely difficult to rein the teenager in, as he or she has grown used to enormous amounts of freedom.

Some social commentators have suggested that many parents have gone too far in the laissez-faire direction, giving children enormous freedom and resources at too young an age – the word 'no' being something they never hear. Indeed, research into parenting styles indicates a trend across many Western countries towards a more laissez-faire parenting style.[13] In old-fashioned language, there is a concern that many children are 'spoilt'. Fortunately, most are not.

Rights *and* responsibilities

As we journey through life our rights and responsibilities gradually grow, in parallel with our competence. As adults we have the right to live where we want, dress how we want, and spend our time and money as we wish. These rights are counterbalanced with responsibilities. We have to work, fulfilling a role in society, in order to get the money we spend. We have a duty to look after our family. We are required to behave in a way that respects the rights of others in our neighbourhood and community.

Parents and other adults working with teenagers must prepare these apprentice adults for both the rights *and* the responsibilities of adulthood. Like all of us, teenagers are keen on their rights. It is important that these are not disconnected from their responsibilities. If we give them all the rights of independent adulthood, without linking them explicitly to an expectation of responsibilities to their community, family and their own futures, we are doing them a disservice.

The increased rights, autonomy and independence that are granted to teenagers should also be connected to their demonstrated competencies. Unfortunately, we sometimes give rights and freedoms to teenagers based simply on their chronological age, rather than assessing their individual ability to manage situations. The argument is made that 'well, he's 16 now, so I just have to let him . . .'. While chronological age provides a decent 'rule of thumb', there is still a need for parents and other adults in mentoring roles to use judgement with the apprentice adult in front of them. If a teenager has demonstrated a relatively poor ability to consistently make decent choices in a particular situation, it is unreasonable to agree to put that teenager into an even more complex and challenging situation just because the teenager 'is at that age'. For example, if a 15-year-old repeatedly gets into difficulty each time he or she is allowed into town with friends, it is unreasonable to allow them to go on an unsupervised camping trip with these friends, even if his or her older brother was permitted to do so when he was 15 years old.

CONCLUSION

Adolescence is a time of enormous change. While the most obvious change is in physical appearance, the most important change is in social skills. Adolescents learn the skills to equip them for independent adult life and so can be conceptualised as apprentice adults. Adolescence is unfairly and unhelpfully caricatured as a time of great and inevitable difficulty. While there can be bumps along that road, most negotiate this phase of lifespan without creating havoc for themselves or their families. As with all phases of the lifespan, there is variability in the pace at which adolescents pick up these new social skills. Brain changes facilitate the acquisition of new skills, as they bring greater problem-solving abilities. School provides an important contained and supportive environment in which adolescents can develop and practise their widening repertoire of social competencies. Adolescents do engage in more risk behaviour than adults, but lack of life experience is perhaps the most important reason underpinning this observation. Parents are a powerful influence on adolescents, and an authoritative parenting style works best.

KEY POINTS

- The primary task of adolescents is learn the skills to manage independent adult life.
- As with others acquiring new competencies or skills, adolescents can be usefully characterised as *apprentice* adults.
- Despite the stereotype, 70% of teenagers experience minimal problems in their adolescent years.
- As with other apprentices, there is inevitable variation among adolescents in the pace and success at which they attain new social skills.
- The brain develops throughout adolescence, with the frontal lobes being last to fully mature, at around 22 years of age.

- While there has been a progressive shift towards more laissez-faire parenting in Western countries recently, authoritative parenting provides the best outcome for adolescents.

REFERENCES

1 Offer D, Schonert-Reichl KA, Boxer AM. Normal adolescent development: empirical research findings. In: Lewis M, editor. *Child and Adolescent Psychiatry: a comprehensive textbook.* 2nd ed. Baltimore, MD: Lippincott, Williams & Wilkins; 1996. pp. 280–90.

2 Shakespeare, W. *A Winter's Tale.* Act III, Scene 3. Oxford: Oxford University Press; 1987.

3 Giedd JN, Blumenthal J, Jeffries NO, *et al.* Brain development during childhood and adolescence: a longitudinal MRI study. *Nat Neurosci.* 1999; **2**(10): 861–3.

4 Blakemore SJ, Choudhury S. Development of the adolescent brain: implications for executive function and social cognition. *J Child Psychol Psychiatry.* 2006; **47**(3–4): 296–312.

5 Piaget J, Inhelder B. *The Growth of Logical Thinking from Childhood to Adolescence: an essay on the construction of formal operational structures.* Oxford: Routledge; 1972.

6 Casey BJ, Jones RM. Neurobiology of the adolescent brain and behavior: implications for substance use disorders. *J Am Acad Child Adolesc Psychiatry.* 2010; **49**(12): 1189–201.

7 Elliott JG. School refusal: issues of conceptualisation, assessment, and treatment. *J Child Psychol Psychiatry.* 2003; **40**(7): 1001–12.

8 Elkind D. Egocentrism in adolescence. *Child Dev.* 1967; **38**(4): 1025–34.

9 McGorry P. Prevention, innovation and implementation science in mental health: the next wave of reform. *Br J Psychiatry.* 2013; **202**(Suppl. 54): S3–4.

10 Baumrind D. Child care practices anteceding three patterns of preschool behaviour. *Genet Psychol Monogr.* 1967; **75**(1): 43–88.

11 Darling N, Steinberg L. Parenting style as context: an integrative model. *Psychol Bull.* 1993; **113**(3): 487–96.

12 Buri JR. Parental authority questionnaire. *J Pers Assess.* 1991; **57**(1): 110–19.

13 Campbell J, Gilmore L. Intergenerational continuities and discontinuities in parenting styles. *Aust J Psychol.* 2007; **59**(3): 140–50.

CHAPTER 3

An overview of substances used by adolescents

INTRODUCTION

Many psychoactive substances are accessible to teenagers today. Alcohol, illegal drugs, illicitly obtained prescribed drugs, and so-called 'head shop' products are readily used. In order to effectively educate and support teenagers, practitioners need a working knowledge of these substances and their effects. This chapter will define and classify various drugs used by teenagers. These drugs will be explored in terms of their effects, risks and prevalence.

WHAT IS A PSYCHOACTIVE DRUG?

Psychoactive drugs are substances that change the user's consciousness, mood or cognitive processes.[1] Essentially, drugs act on areas of the brain that regulate a person's mood, thoughts and motivations. Psychoactive drugs can be legal or illegal and can be used for medical, recreational and spiritual reasons.

Classification of psychoactive drugs

Psychoactive drugs can be classified in a number of ways. Perhaps the simplest way is to consider their effect. Notably, some drugs, such as cannabis, have properties that are evident in more than one category. Later in this chapter, we will examine the most commonly used depressants, stimulants and hallucinogens.

BOX 3.1 Central nervous system depressants

Central nervous system (CNS) depressants are drugs with a sedating effect. The physiological effect is one of slowing down, bringing on drowsiness or putting the user to sleep. Alcohol and cannabis are commonly used depressant drugs.

BOX 3.2 Central nervous system stimulants

Stimulants do exactly what they say, they stimulate the CNS. Adolescents who use them experience a sense of speeding up, high energy levels and elevated alertness. Cocaine is an example of a CNS stimulant.

BOX 3.3 Hallucinogens

Hallucinogens alter the perceptions of the user. Visual or auditory hallucinations occur. The user may experience things that aren't really happening and can find his or her reality is completely or partially distorted. LSD, commonly referred to as acid, is perhaps the best-known hallucinogen.

TABLE 3.1 Commonly used drugs classified by effect

CNS depressants	CNS stimulants	Hallucinogens
Alcohol	Amphetamine	LSD
General anaesthetics	Ecstasy	Magic mushrooms
Benzodiazepines	Cocaine	Peyote
Inhalants	Crack cocaine	Ibogagaine
Synthetic hypnotics	Caffeine	Salvia
Opiates and opioids	Nicotine	
Cannabis	Mephedrone	

Drug use results in a psychoactive effect because it alters the activity of neurotransmitters within the brain. There are many neurotransmitters that permit communication from one brain cell or neuron to the next. Some neurotransmitters increase electric activity in neurons, while others inhibit activity. The brain pathway involved in drug use is the reward pathway, deep in the limbic system. Activity in this pathway is increased naturally by pleasurable behaviours such as eating nice food or sexual activity. The main neurotransmitter in the reward pathway is dopamine. Virtually, every psychoactive drug listed in Table 3.1 causes increased dopamine activity in this reward pathway, thereby inducing pleasurable feelings.

BASIC PHARMACOLOGY

To understand any drug, we must consider basic pharmacology. Four primary factors influence the effect of psychoactive substances.[2]
1 Route of administration (ROA)
2 Distribution
3 Interaction
4 Elimination

Route of administration

ROA refers to how drugs enter the body and the bloodstream. It is linked to the risk the drug poses. For example, injecting heroin is riskier than smoking it, as a larger quantity gets into the bloodstream more quickly. This makes the effects more potent and overdoses more likely. ROA influences how quickly the drug takes effect and impacts on how addictive it is. Some drugs are administered in more than one way, whereas others will only work with particular ROAs. *See* Table 3.2 for further information.

Distribution

The circulation and accumulation of the drug through the body is known as distribution. It governs how much of the substance is accessible to the brain. For example, cannabis is fat-soluble and is distributed to more of the body than other drugs, and will stay in the system longer.

Interaction

Interaction relates to the way in which the drug interacts with other drugs the user takes. Many adolescents use numerous substances at a time. Drugs can interact with each other in three ways.
1 They add to each other's effects, becoming toxic (e.g. alcohol exacerbates the respiratory depression caused by heroin).
2 They interfere with the actions of other drugs, sometimes cancelling out another drug's effects. For example, benzodiazepines counteract the stimulant effect of amphetamine, allowing the user to sleep 'when the party is over'.
3 A new drug is created from the interaction of two other drugs (e.g. alcohol and cocaine result in creation of cocaethylene).

TABLE 3.2 Common routes of administration[3]

Route of administration	Description	Advantages	Disadvantages
Oral administration	Taken by mouth	Easy to do Slow onset of action (15–30 minutes on an empty stomach) 75% absorbed in 1–3 hours	Stomach distress Food may delay absorption Some drugs are destroyed in the stomach
Inhalation	Drawing psychoactive substances into the lungs with the breath (e.g. smoking)	Almost instant onset of action Can be used when person experiences stomach distress	Can't control dose Almost instant onset of action Irritation of respiratory system
Absorption through the mucous membranes	Drug is administered through mucous membranes (nose, mouth, throat, vagina, rectum, eyes), e.g. snorting or sucking/dissolving in the mouth	Rapid onset of action	Dose control is difficult Mucous membranes can become irritated
Parenteral injections: IV IM SubQ	IV is an injection into the vein IM is an injection into a muscle mass SubQ is an injection under the skin (sometimes called 'skin popping')	Rapid onset of action Some drugs can be injected that can't be swallowed because of irritation	Irritation/infection of tissue (abscesses) Poor injecting technique (injection into an artery or nerve) Painful to some people Transmission of blood-borne viruses when paraphernalia shared

Note: IV, intravenous injection; IM, intramuscular injection; SubQ, subcutaneous injection

Elimination

Elimination is how the substance leaves the body. Initially, the liver breaks down most drugs into component parts, called metabolites. Metabolites are chemicals that are usually less psychoactive than the original drugs. Following this, the kidneys are the major routes of elimination via urine.

When discussing elimination, we must remember that certain drugs are eliminated from the body quicker than others. Cannabis, benzodiazepines and heroin all remain in the body for days, if not weeks, after someone takes them. Other substances such as alcohol, cocaine and ecstasy are eliminated much more quickly. This variation in the elimination of different substances has important implications when it comes to drug screening (*see* Chapter 11).

Other factors to consider

Other factors can affect the drug effect. The purity of the substance, the speed of administration, and the user's physiology all play a role. If two people ingest 6 units of alcohol but one is a small, slim, adolescent female who drinks 6 units in an hour on an empty stomach and the other is a grown man who drinks the 6 units over a 6-hour period after eating dinner, these two people will experience a different effect.

Why are some drugs more addictive than others?

Research indicates that the addictiveness of a drug is linked to its ability to induce a rapid increase in dopamine activity. For example, coca leaves contain cocaine. When chewed the chemical enters the bloodstream slowly, and gradually increases dopamine activity. This induces a slight sense of pleasure. When the same drug is injected or snorted, the blood concentration goes from zero to a high level within seconds. This causes an instantaneous surge in dopamine activity, which is experienced as intensely pleasurable. Figure 3.1 presents this diagrammatically. The addictiveness of the behaviour is determined by the steepness of the curve as it moves upwards.

Methadone and heroin both stimulate the opiate receptor, which ultimately increases dopamine activity. However, a person is much more likely to abuse injected heroin than oral methadone, as the former behaviour causes a much more rapid change in dopamine activity.

COMMONLY USED SUBSTANCES

Alcohol

Alcohol is an intoxicating beverage made by fermenting sugar and plant materials. The active ingredient is ethyl alcohol. Alcohol is a CNS depressant. There is substantial international variation in measures of alcohol. In the UK, a measure

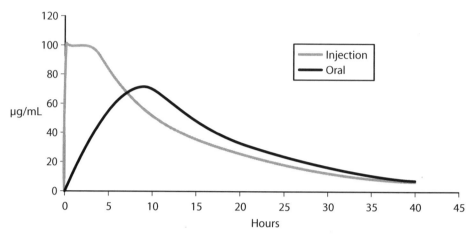

FIGURE 3.1 Change in blood concentration of drug following oral and injected administration

is called a 'unit', while in other locations it is called a 'standard drink'. This variability in language contributes to confusion among both professionals and the public. One UK unit of alcohol is measured as 10 mL or 8 g of pure alcohol.[4] It takes the body about 1 hour to eliminate 10 mL of alcohol. Alcohol is typically consumed as wine, beer and spirits such as whisky and vodka. However, some people make their own alcohol, such as poteen in Ireland. There is evidence of people drinking products that contain alcohol but were not made for human consumption, such as aftershave and methylated spirits. Naturally, this is worrying but thankfully rare among adolescents.

BOX 3.4 Guidelines on low-risk drinking for adults

- *Adult males*: no more than 210 mL of pure alcohol (i.e. 21 UK units) per week and no more than 40 mL in any one day.
- *Adult females*: no more than 140 mL of pure alcohol (i.e. 14 UK units) per week and no more than 30 mL in any one day.
- *Adolescents*: there are no agreed guidelines on levels of drinking that can be considered low risk to people under 18 years of age.

Routes of administration
The normal method of administration for alcohol is to drink it.

Drug effects
The effect of alcohol depends on the amount taken. Although alcohol is a depressant, it can have a stimulating effect. Common effects following

consumption include a sense of dis-inhibition, social freedom and excitement, the proverbial 'Dutch courage', and a warm feeling of enjoyment.[5] At higher doses alcohol can affect the cerebellum, which results in poor balance and slurred speech.

Side effects

Some commonly experienced side effects from alcohol include:

- increased heart rate
- dilated blood vessels – flushed skin
- increased need to urinate
- increased sweating
- hangover
- poor motor coordination
- vomiting
- blackouts
- incontinence
- difficulty performing sexually.

Risks of use

Adolescents are more sensitive to alcohol and may not have the same tolerance as adults. As they are still developing physically, the risk of harm may be increased. Adolescent alcohol use may result in long-term effects on the brain, on bone maturation, and on the reproductive system. Alcohol is a contributing factor in more than 60 medical conditions such as liver disease, heart problems, cancer, pancreatitis and stomach problems.[6,7]

Alcohol is strongly associated with a range of social problems such as violence, mental health concerns, suicidality, family problems, and accidental death. Heavy drinking in adolescence leads to later harm.[8] Often adolescents under the influence of alcohol will be clumsier than they would be sober. Falls, accidents and fights often occur. In countries such as Britain, Ireland and Australia, visit any hospital emergency department at the weekend and you will see evidence of this side effect.

Regular use results in *tolerance*. Essentially, the person needs more alcohol to achieve the same level of intoxication. Daily use over a prolonged period can result in withdrawal symptoms when the person stops drinking. These are physically and psychologically unpleasant, and can be dangerous (e.g. withdrawal seizures).

Prevalence

TABLE 3.3 Alcohol Prevalence Rates[9-11]

Age (years)	Europe	England/UK	Ireland	Australia
15–16	87% lifetime	90% lifetime	81% lifetime	
	79% past year	85% past year	73% past year	
	57% past month	65% past month	50% past month	
11–15		21% past week		
12–17				80% lifetime
				23% past week

Cannabis

Cannabis is derived from the cannabis plant. Its active ingredient is THC. Cannabis comes in three forms.

1 Cannabis resin (hash) is a brown/black lump made from compressed resin of the plant. It comes in 9 oz bars (referred to as nine bars), which are cut into smaller 'deals' and sold.
2 Weed is dried parts of the plant. It comes in a small bag containing the loose herb. With modern hydroponic growing techniques, selective removal of male plants and cross breeding of cannabis strains, the concentration of THC has increased greatly in the past 40 years, from about 3% to up to 20%.
3 Hash oil is the strongest form. It ranges from amber to dark brown in colour and current samples contain anything from 15% to 70% THC. One to two drops of this oil on a cigarette is equal to smoking a joint.[12]

Routes of administration

Cannabis can be smoked with tobacco in a rolled cigarette (joint or spliff); it can be smoked in raw form in a pipe (bong) and it can be eaten (e.g. brownie). It can also be heated in a vaporiser. This latter method has the advantage of avoiding the inhalation of potentially carcinogenic smoke.

Drug effects

Because cannabis is usually smoked, the drug effect is rapid. Getting 'stoned' gives a feeling of relaxation, mild euphoria and makes the person talkative.[13] Users may experience a state of detached observation and increased appetite ('the munchies').[13] Some users describe increased appreciation of colours and sound, and changes in perceptions of time and space.[5,14]

Side effects

Users can experience a range of unpleasant effects, including:

- red eyes
- elevated heart rate
- acute anxiety
- delusion
- hallucinations
- paranoia

- increased self-consciousness
- changes in blood pressure
- dry mouth
- increased appetite
- tiredness
- nausea and vomiting.[13]

Risks of use

While some argue that cannabis is relatively safe, there are risks. Smoking large amounts combined, in many cases, with tobacco increases the risk of cancer and heart disease. Cannabis interferes with one's ability to concentrate and control motor coordination; therefore, driving or operating machinery under the influence can increase risk of an accident.[13] Regular cannabis use is linked with an array of mental health problems.[15] Individuals with existing mental health concerns may find that cannabis use triggers schizophrenia or psychosis. One recent study found that adolescents who use cannabis are twice as likely to develop psychosis by the time they reach young adulthood than those who don't.[16]

Cannabis use is associated with lasting deficits in attention and working memory.[17] An increase in educational underachievement, leaving school early, failure to attend third-level education and failure to attain a degree are all associated with its use.[18] Motivation can be affected by ongoing use. While withdrawal symptoms are not as pronounced as in other drugs, some troubling withdrawals do occur with sudden cessation of regular use. The most common symptoms include insomnia, vivid dreams and irritability.

Prevalence

TABLE 3.4 Cannabis prevalence rates[9,11]

Age (years)	Europe	UK	Ireland	Australia
15–16	17% lifetime 13% past year 7% past month	25% lifetime 21% past year 13% past month	18% lifetime 14% past year 7% past month	
12–15				19% lifetime 4.3% past month 2.6% past week
16–17				24.6% lifetime 10.9% past month 5.9% past week

Cocaine

Cocaine is a powerful CNS stimulant derived from the South American *Erythroxylon coca* plant. It comes in two forms: cocaine hyrdrochloride, a white powder, and crack cocaine, off-white crystal rocks that have been processed to remove the hydrochloride so that it can be smoked. The effects of cocaine powder can last up to 30 minutes, whereas crack gives a shorter but more intense high.

Routes of administration

Cocaine hydrochloride can be snorted, gummed or injected. Snorting and intravenous are the most common ROA. Crack is smoked in a crack pipe. It gets its name from the crackling noise it makes when heated.

Drug effects

The effects of cocaine include a feeling of intense euphoria, a sense of invincibility, hyper-alertness, high confidence, increased energy levels, appetite suppression, and an overall feeling of exhilaration.

Side effects

Cocaine has numerous undesirable side effects, including:

- restlessness
- agitation
- paranoia
- palpitations
- increased heart rate
- increased body temperature
- breathing problems (crack lung)
- sores on mouth
- sweating
- headaches
- nosebleeds
- irritability
- aggression
- depression
- exhaustion
- deviated septum.

Risks of use

Cocaine users are at risk for a range of social, medical and relational problems. As with any intravenous drug use, sharing equipment increases risk of transmitting viruses. However, sharing straws and notes for snorting cocaine, and sharing pipes for smoking cocaine is also risky in terms of contracting HIV or hepatitis. Difficulty achieving an orgasm, and low sperm count in men can be a consequence and some women experience difficulties with menstruation.

Because cocaine contracts blood vessels, users are at risk of clots. Heart attacks, strokes and kidney failure are associated with cocaine use. Overdose can occur and the risk increases when cocaine is mixed with alcohol or other drugs. Cocaine can have a detrimental effect on mental health. At autopsy, it's not uncommon to find cocaine in the systems of suicide victims.[19] Some people can develop psychosis, which may include violent behaviour. Cocaine use is related to intentional injuries (homicide, suicide, non-fatal injury) and injuries in general.[20]

Prevalence

TABLE 3.5 Cocaine prevalence rates[9,11,21,22]

Age (years)	Europe	UK	Ireland	Australia
15–16	2% lifetime (cocaine) 2% lifetime (crack)	5% lifetime (cocaine) 2% lifetime (crack)	3% lifetime (cocaine) 2% lifetime (crack)	
12–15				1.9% lifetime
16–17				3.7% lifetime
16–24		10.8% lifetime (cocaine)	6.3% lifetime (cocaine) 1.5% lifetime (crack)	

Heroin and the opioids

Heroin is in the opioid drug family. This drug family includes natural opiates such as morphine and synthetic opioids such as dihydrocodeine. Opiates are powerful painkillers. Heroin is derived from morphine and is stronger than opium or morphine. On the street, it usually comes in the form of a brown powder.

Routes of administration

Heroin can be injected or smoked. Most heroin users 'smoke' the drug initially. Users create a foil tray and a tube (tooter) and heat the tray with a cigarette lighter so the heroin 'runs' in lines. The vapour is inhaled through the tube. This is what gave name to the colloquialism 'chasing the dragon', as the user is literally chasing the vapour rising from the foil. Some heroin users progress to injecting, especially if they have become dependent on the drug. Heroin is not water-soluble and in order to inject it, it is broken down with acid. In many needle exchange facilities, intravenous users are given kits commonly referred to as 'works' that include sterile water, citric acid, filters and clean needles. Heroin is usually injected directly into a vein (intravenously), although users new to injecting sometimes inject subcutaneously (skin-popping) or into a muscle (intramuscularly) first. Subcutaneous and intramuscular injecting is more likely to lead to infections. Less common ROAs include snorting and smoking it in a cigarette or a cannabis joint.

Abuse of prescription opioids is a major problem in some countries. They can come in injection and liquid and tablet forms. Some users will crush up tablets for injection. However, the risk of infection is high with this. Methadone, a replacement drug used to treat opiate addiction, usually comes in liquid form and it is drunk on a daily basis. Taking any opiate, particularly when someone has not developed a tolerance for it can be dangerous and lead to a potentially fatal overdose.

Drug effects

Heroin, when injected, produces an initial rush of excitement followed by a peaceful, dreamlike state. Users report feeling relaxed, drowsy and warm.[15] Opiates relieve pain and distress and create a sense of detachment.[5]

Side effects

Heroin is a CNS depressant, and while someone is under the influence, their pupils will be constricted (pinned), they may nod off repeatedly ('goofing off', 'on the nod'), and their speech may be slower and slurred. Other common side effects include:

- reduced sex drive
- slowing of major organ systems
- low blood pressure
- mensturation ceasing
- decreased respiration
- decreased heart rate and blood pressure
- constipation
- nausea/vomiting.

Risks of use

Physical addiction is a risk with regular use. Nearly 25% of people who use heroin become addicted.[23] Withdrawal is unpleasant but rarely dangerous. Common symptoms include sweating, vomiting, diarrhoea, cramps, muscular pains, sleep disturbance, hot flushes and psychological distress. Objectively, the symptoms are like a bad dose of the flu; however, when coupled with the anxiety, depressive symptoms, difficulty sleeping and the loss of the primary drug effect of euphoria, the symptoms are amplified.

Risk of overdose is high, particularly in users without a tolerance and those returning to use after a period of abstinence. The risk is increased when users take other CNS depressants in conjunction with heroin. The risk of transmitting HIV and hepatitis B and C is high for intravenous users who share using paraphernalia. Street heroin is commonly mixed with a range of ingredients (e.g. sugar, talc, other drugs) and soft tissue infection is common. Abscesses, cellulitis, and even gangrene can occur. Collapsed veins are another common problem.

Prevalence

TABLE 3.6 Heroin prevalence rates[5,11,15]

Age (years)	Europe	UK	Ireland	Australia
15–16	1% lifetime (heroin)	2% lifetime (heroin)	1% lifetime (heroin)	
12–15				2% lifetime (opiates)
16–17				2.3% lifetime (opiates)

Ecstasy

Ecstasy is a man-made drug containing the ingredient MDMA. It is sold in tablet form in varying colours, with various symbols etched on the surface (e.g. dove, smiley face). These symbols frequently give them their names. It has both stimulant and hallucinogenic properties. It is used in dance clubs and raves as well as a variety of other settings.

Routes of administration

Ecstasy is usually taken orally in tablet form, however some users report using powered MDMA.

Drug effects

Ecstasy is a stimulant. It generates feelings of empathy and is referred to as 'the love drug'.[5] Ecstasy can heighten perceptual experience. Sounds, colours and emotions feel more intense.[15] Users feel more alert, confident and energetic.[24] People who use ecstasy also report intense skin tingles (rushes). A desire to be close to others, to touch and to use the created energy is often experienced.

Side effects

Common side effects of ecstasy include:

- dilated pupils
- jaw clenching
- increased body temperature
- sweating
- nausea/vomiting

- palpitations
- confusion and exhaustion
- dehydration
- sleep disturbance
- low mood

- increased blood pressure
- increased heart rate
- paranoia ('freaking out')
- convulsions
- aggression
- lowered inhibitions.[15,24,25]

Risks of use

Deaths from ecstasy are rare. When they occur, they can be attributed to heat stroke, heart attacks and brain haemorrhage.[15,24] In high doses, MDMA can interfere with the body's ability to regulate temperature. On rare but unpredictable occasions, this leads to a sharp increase in body temperature (hyperthermia), which results in liver, kidney, cardiovascular system failure or death.[25]

As ecstasy is a synthetic drug, there is no regulation on dose and no way of knowing what it is mixed with. Animal research suggests that even short-term use can lead to long-term damage on the brain's pleasure pathways. Many users describe the 'come down' as difficult. It is characterised by low mood, difficulty sleeping, aches and pains, anxiety, paranoia and exhaustion.[24] Those taking ecstasy sometimes take CNS depressants such as benzodiazepines to help them relax. Anecdotally, heroin users often report that their first instance of heroin occurred while they were coming down off ecstasy. Ecstasy users report a myriad of social problems including financial, relationship and occupational problems.[26] While ecstasy can increase sexual desire, it also impairs sexual functioning.[27,28]

Prevalence

TABLE 3.7 Ecstasy prevalence rates[9-11,22]

Age (years)	Europe	UK	Ireland	Australia
15–16	3% lifetime 2% past year 1% past month	4% lifetime 3% past year 1% past month	2% lifetime 2% past year 1% past month	
12–15				2.5% lifetime
16–17				7.8% lifetime
16–24		10.4% lifetime	6.5% lifetime	

Benzodiazepines and 'Z' drugs

Benzodiazepines are CNS depressant medications prescribed for a range of medical and psychiatric problems. Benzodiazepines are used to treat anxiety and sleep disturbance. They are also used in treating alcohol withdrawal, seizures and as a muscle relaxant. The most well-known benzodiazepines include diazepam (valium, anxicalm), alprazolam (Xanax, Gerax), flurazepam

(Dalmane), flunitrazepam (Rohypnol), and chlordiazepoxide (Librium). The 'Z' drugs (zolpidem and zopiclone) are a related group of medications that are used as sleeping tablets.

In view of the popularity of these drugs, there is increasing trade in benzodiazepines on the Internet. When abused, people can consume enormous amounts of these drugs each day. Some users may report consuming many multiples of the normally prescribed dose.

Routes of administration

Benzodiazepines come in tablet or capsule form and the normal ROA is oral. Some users crush them, or open capsules and inject it. Some benzodiazepines are available as liquids and in injectable forms, or as suppositories for rectal administration, as made famous by Ewan McGregor in *Trainspotting*.

Drug effects

When people misuse benzodiazepines they are seeking a calming feeling. With high doses, disinhibition occurs. Some users report a feeling of being in a bubble. People 'coming down' off stimulant drugs such as ecstasy and cocaine sometimes use them to relieve the unpleasantness of the come-down.

Side effects

There are many side effects to benzodiazepine use. 'Blackouts' are common. Depending on tolerance level and dose, users may experience the following:

- blurred vision
- dense amnesia
- impaired thinking
- drowsiness
- dry mouth
- slurred speech
- muscle weakness
- disinhibition
- shakiness
- impaired motor coordination
- nausea and vomiting
- diarrhoea or constipation
- tiredness and reduced alertness
- difficulty feeling emotions.

Benzodiazepines can have a paradoxical effect. Rather than making you feel calm, they can bring about feelings of restlessness, irritability and rage. They can lead to hallucinations, loss of self-control and nightmares.

Risks of use

Benzodiazepines can produce physical dependence. Withdrawals are unpleasant and benzodiazepine withdrawal may include the following symptoms:

- anxiety
- sleep disturbance
- aggression
- weakness
- seizures
- unsteady gait
- feeling ground is moving
- depression
- hallucinations
- paranoia
- restlessness
- pain
- confusion
- nausea/cramps
- depersonalisation.[29]

Overdose is relatively common. However, when benzodiazepines are taken alone, even in large doses, there is a low risk of fatality. Fatal overdoses usually occur where these drugs are mixed with other depressants (e.g. alcohol, heroin, methadone).[30] Benzodiazepine use is associated with accidents and falls (particularly in the elderly).[5] When the benzodiazepines that come in tablet form are crushed up and injected, the risk of infection, cellulitis and abscesses increases.

Prevalence

It is difficult to accurately estimate the percentage of adolescents using benzodiazepines as most national and international surveys vary how they ask this question. In the majority of studies into prevalence rates, tranquillisers, sedatives and sleeping pills are lumped in together.

TABLE 3.8 Prevalence rates of tranquillisers/sedatives[9,11,22]

Age (years)	Europe	UK	Ireland	Australia
15–16	6% lifetime	2% lifetime	3% lifetime	
12–15				16.2% lifetime
16–17				19% lifetime
16–24			4.8% lifetime	

Amphetamines

Amphetamines are CNS stimulants. Two common forms are amphetamine (speed) and methamphetamine (crystal meth). Amphetamines usually come in powder form (speed) and as small crystal 'rocks'. There are medical uses for amphetamines, such as the treatment of attention deficit hyperactivity disorder and narcolepsy.

Routes of administration

Amphetamines can be swallowed, snorted, injected or smoked. Methamphetamine is most commonly smoked in a glass pipe.

Drug effects

Amphetamines create alertness, energy and excitement. Users can experience a sense of superiority, well-being, cleverness and competence.[31,32] Amphetamines decrease the need for sleep and are sometimes abused by exam students. Methamphetamine causes a release of dopamine and serotonin, giving users an intense rush of pleasure.

Side effects

There are multitudes of side effects to amphetamine use, including:

- shakes
- high blood pressure
- increased heart rate
- blurred vision
- dizziness
- agitation
- anxiety
- repetition of behaviour
- sweating
- headaches
- paranoia hallucinations
- nausea/cramps
- hostility and aggression
- dry mouth
- palpitations
- difficulty breathing
- mood swings
- raised temperature.

Risks of use

Amphetamines can lead to a drug-induced psychosis. This manifests in a presentation mirroring schizophrenia. Rapid weight loss is seen in regular users. The impact on sleep can be enormous. Sleep disturbance, coupled with weight loss and reduced appetite can lead to being run down. Teeth grinding and jaw clenching are common side effects. Dental problems, cracked teeth and poor hygiene are common. The high blood pressure and irregular heart rate can stress the heart, leading to increased risk of cardiac arrest.

Amphetamines are associated with risky sexual behaviours, unplanned pregnancy and sexually transmitted infections. Because of the aggression frequently seen, social and forensic risks are increased. Relationship, family and legal problems are common.

For regular users, going without sleep poses a risk of paranoia and aggression. On the street, this is known as 'tweaking'. The lack of sleep, intense craving for methamphetamine and frustration caused by being unable to achieve the original high can result in violent behaviour, extreme irrationality, paranoia and spur-of-the-moment crime.[33] Practitioners are advised to be extremely careful when dealing with someone who is tweaking.

Prevalence

TABLE 3.9 Amphetamine prevalence rates[9-11,22]

Age (years)	Europe	UK	Ireland	Australia
15–16	3% lifetime	4% lifetime	2% lifetime	
12–15				2.6% lifetime
16–17				6.2% lifetime
16–24		11.3% lifetime	3.2% lifetime	

Volatiles

Volatiles comprise substances that contain gas or volatile liquid. Commonly abused volatiles include pressurised sprays such as deodorants, some glues, paint thinners, various pressurised gases and petrol.

Routes of administration

The ROA is inhalation. The substances are inhaled directly from their container or sprayed/poured into a bag. 'Huffing' refers to the practice of soaking a cloth with the chemical and holding it to the face.

Drug effects

The psychoactive effect of inhalants is similar to alcohol. Initially, there is a short feeling of stimulation. Users then experience a sense of intoxication, dreaminess, drowsiness and a lowering of inhibitions.

Side effects

The side effects of volatiles are plentiful and unpleasant. They include:

- headaches and nausea
- muscle weakness
- abdominal pain
- severe mood swings
- violent behaviour
- belligerence
- slurred speech
- numbness of the extremities
- visual disturbances
- limb spasms
- lack of coordination
- apathy/lethargy
- impaired judgement
- depressed reflexes
- loss of consciousness
- hearing loss.[34]

Risks of use

Volatile use is unpredictable and dangerous. There is no safe way to take them.

The greatest risk is 'sudden sniffing death syndrome'. Young people tend to use these substances in a place where they won't be discovered, which increases risk of accidental death. Suffocation, death following aspiration of vomit and spasm of the larynx can also occur.[5]

Other consequences include liver and kidney damage, hearing loss, CNS damage and harm to bone marrow. Long-term users can experience weight loss, mood disorders, disorientation and difficulty concentrating. Sniffing can cause a progressive decline in cognitive functioning that may lead to permanent neurological changes.[35] Impairments in processing speed, sustained attention, memory retrieval and language can all occur with volatile use.[36]

Prevalence

TABLE 3.10 Volatiles prevalence rates[9-11,22]

Age (years)	Europe	UK	Ireland	Australia
15–16	9% lifetime	10% lifetime	9% lifetime	
	5% past year	7% past year	5% past year	
	2% past month	3% past month	2% past month	
12–17				18.7% lifetime
				13.5% past year
				7.9% past month
16–24		3.6% lifetime	5.9% lifetime	

NOVEL PSYCHOACTIVE SUBSTANCES: 'LEGAL HIGHS' AND HEAD SHOP DRUGS

In recent years, we have seen synthetic and 'herbal' products flood the market. For the purpose of this book, they are referred to as novel psychoactive substances (NPSs). Up until recently, no laws were in place to stop the sale of these 'legal highs.' Vendors bypassed narcotics, medicine and food product legislation by selling them as 'bath salts' or 'plant food'. Despite new legislation in many countries, many NPSs are still available on the street or online. It would be impossible, in the scope of this book, to discuss each one. However, NPSs can be loosely categorised into three classes:

1 NPSs that are smoked
2 NPSs that are snorted
3 NPSs that are taken in tablet form, party pills.[37]

1 NPSs that are smoked

Common substances include Spice and *Salvia divinorum*. Spice products contain one of a number of synthetic cannabinoids. This chemical is sprayed onto dried plant material. Salvia is a cannabis alternative that comes from the salvia plant. These products are sold as smokeable herbal mixtures. Salvia is a widely used NPS. There is limited research on the harmful effects of NPSs, but in a recent Irish study, respondents linked its use to headaches, mental health problems, depression and antisocial behaviour.[38]

2 NPSs that are snorted

Mephedrone is a NSP used as an alternative to amphetamines. Mephedrone is derived from cathinone, the active ingredient in the khat plant. Although mephedrone is usually consumed via snorting, there is some intravenous use in long-term heroin users. It can also be swallowed in capsules or as powder wrapped up in a cigarette paper.

Mephedrone use carries risk of aggression, anxiety, psychosis and hallucinations.[39–41] Intravenous use brings with it a whole gamut of problems. It carries greater risk of local tissue infection, abscesses and even gangrene than other injected drugs. For those who share using paraphernalia, risk of transmitting a blood-borne virus is present. Agitation, tachycardia, hypertension and seizures are also reported as side effects.[42]

3 NPSs that are taken in tablet form, party pills

Benzlpiperazine, or BZP, has been listed as a controlled substance in the European Union; however, many other amphetamine-like substances were created and sold as 'party pills'. These NPSs, close in chemical structure to amphetamines, are thought to have similar effects. Users can experience sleep disturbance, nausea and vomiting, difficulty urinating and seizures. Hallucinations, paranoia and depression are also reported.[43]

CONCLUSION

Having a good understanding of the substances used by adolescents is important. Each substance carries with it its own effects, side effects and consequences. The ability to discuss, educate and support young people around substance use is a vital skill needed by practitioners. Being able to talk the same language and understand the effects of substances will open lines of communication between worker and young person. You won't know everything about every drug. One way to find out more is to ask the young person you are working with. Often teenagers are happy to discuss the drug, how they take it and the effects it has on them. This can be a good way of building a relationship, getting an insight into their situation and learning more about drugs in general.

KEY POINTS

- A variety of drugs are available. Over time patterns and popularity of particular drugs vary.
- Drugs can be considered in three categories: CNS stimulants, CNS depressants and hallucinogens.
- All drugs have unique effects and these vary depending on how the drug is consumed.
- Alcohol and cannabis are by far the most commonly used substances by teens around the world.

RESOURCES

Various websites provide a wealth of information in relation to various drugs. The following are some of the most useful:

- National Institute on Drug Abuse (www.drugabuse.gov)
- Drugs.i.e. (www.drugs.i.e.)
- National Cannabis Prevention and Information Centre (www.ncpic.org.au)
- Global Drugs Survey (www.globaldrugsurvey.com)
- Centre for Addiction and Mental Health (www.camh.net).

FURTHER READING

➡ Peterson T. *Working with Substance Misusers: a guide to theory and practice.* London: Routledge; 2005.

REFERENCES

1 World Health Organization (WHO). *Neuroscience of Psychoactive Substance Use and Dependence.* Geneva: WHO; 2004.
2 Radcliffe AB, Cruse J, Rush PA. *The Pharmer's Almanac: the pharmacology of drugs.* San Francisco, CA: MAC Printing and Publications; 1985.
3 Cox JR. *Pharmacology and Biopharmaceutics Learner's Handbook.* Minneapolis, MN: International Addiction Counsellor Training Programme; 2003.
4 Erithacus. *Commentary on the Measurement Muddle in the UK.* Metric Views; 2007 [Cited 18 January 2007]. Available at: http://metricviews.org.uk/2007/01/units-of-alcohol/
5 McBride A. Some drugs of misuse. In: Peterson T, McBride A, editors. *Working with Substance Misusers: a guide to theory and practice.* London: Routledge; 2005. pp. 3–22.
6 World Health Organization (WHO). *Global Health Risks: mortality and burden of disease attributable to selected major risks.* Geneva: WHO; 2009.
7 Talktofrank.com [Internet]. London: c2011 [Cited 16 October 2011]. Available at: www.talktofrank.com/drug/alcohol

8 International Centre for Alcohol Policies. Module 11. Young people and alcohol. Washington, DC; 2005 [Cited 8 February 2013]. Available at: www.icap.org/portals/0/download/all_pdfs/blue_book/Module_11_Young_People_and_Alcohol.pdf

9 Hibell B, Guttormsson U, Ahlström S, *et al*. *The 2011 ESPAD Report: substance use among students in 36 European Countries*. Stockholm: The Swedish Council for Information on Alcohol and Other Drugs (CAN); 2012.

10 National Health Service (NHS). *Statistics on Alcohol in England*. London: The Information Centre, NHS; 2007.

11 White V, Smith G. *Australian Secondary Students' Use of Over-The-Counter and Illicit Substances in 2008*. Melbourne: Cancer Council Victoria; 2008.

12 Streetdrugs.org [Cited 8 February 2013]. Available at: www.streetdrugs.org/html%20files/Hash%20Oil.html

13 Boyce A, McArdle P. Long-term effects of cannabis. *Paediatr Child Health*. 2008; **18**(1): 37–41.

14 Health Service Executive. *Know the Facts about Drugs*. Dublin: Health Promotion Unit; 2008.

15 Griffith-Lendering MFH, Huijbregts SCH, Mooijaart A, *et al*. Cannabis use and development of externalising and internalising behaviour problems in early adolescence. *Drug Alcohol Depend*. 2011; **116**(1–3): 11–17.

16 Arseneault L, Cannon M, Poulton R. Causal association between cannabis and psychosis: examination of the evidence. *Br J Psychiatry*. 2004; **184**: 110–17.

17 Rubino T, Parolaro D. Long lasting consequences of cannabis exposure in adolescence. *Mol Cell Endocrinol*. 2008; **286**(1–2 Suppl. 1): S108–13.

18 Horwood LJ, Fergusson DM, Hayatbakhsh MR, *et al*. Cannabis use and educational achievement: findings from three Australasian cohort studies. *Drug Alcohol Depend*. 2010; **110**: 247–53.

19 Centers for Disease Control and Prevention (CDC). Toxicology testing and results for suicide victims; 13 states, 2004. *MMWR Morb Mortal Wkly Rep*. 2006; **55**(46): 1245–8.

20 Macdonald S, Anglin-Bodrug K, Mann RE, *et al*. Injury risk associated with cannabis and cocaine use. *Drug Alcohol Depend*. 2003; **72**(2): 99–115.

21 Diment E, Harris J, Jotangia D, *et al*. *Smoking, Drinking and Drug Use Among Young People in England in 2008*. Leeds: The Information Centre; 2009.

22 National Advisory Committee on Drugs. *Drug Use in Ireland and Northern Ireland 2006/2007: drug prevalence survey bulletin 2*. Dublin: Regional Drug Task Force (Ireland) and Health and Social Services Board (Northern Ireland); 2008.

23 National Institute on Drug Abuse. *Heroin: info facts pamphlet*. Bethesda, MD: National Institute on Drug Abuse; 2010.

24 Druginfo.adf.org.au [Internet]. Melbourne: Australian Drug Foundation; c2011. [Updated 4 February 2011; Cited 16 October 2011]. Available at: www.druginfo.adf.org.au/index.php?option=com_content&view=article&id=394&Itemid=50

25 National Institute on Drug Abuse. *Ecstasy: info facts pamphlet*. Bethesda, MD: National Institute on Drug Abuse; 2010.

26 Topp L, Hando J, Dillon P, *et al*. Ecstasy use in Australia: patterns of use and associate harm. *Drug Alcohol Depend*. 1999; **55**(1–2): 105–15.

27 Zeimishlany Z, Aizenberg D, Wiezman A. Subjective effects of MDMA (Ecstasy) on human sexual function. *Eur Psychiatry.* 2001; **16**(2): 127–30.

28 Passie T, Harmann U, Schneider U, *et al.* Ecstasy (MDMA) mimics the post-orgasmic state: impairment of sexual drive and function during acute MDMA-effects may be due to increased prolactin secretion. *Med Hypotheses.* 2005; **64**(5): 899–903.

29 Healy D. *Psychiatric Drugs Explained.* 4th ed. London: Churchill Livingstone; 2005.

30 Nurses' Health Promotion Committee. *Benzodiazepine Misuse.* Dublin: Nursing Health Promotion Initiative, Addiction Services, Health Service Executive; 2010.

31 Centre for Addiction and Mental Health. *Do you Know . . . Amphetamines.* Toronto: Centre for Addiction and Mental Health; 2004.

32 Centre for Substance Abuse Research. *Amphetamines.* College Park: University of Maryland. Available at: www.cesar.umd.edu/cesar/drugs/amphetamines.asp (accessed 19 October 2011).

33 Centre for Substance Abuse Research. *Methamphetamines.* College Park: University of Maryland [Cited 19 October 2011.] Available at: www.cesar.umd.edu/cesar/drugs/meth.asp

34 Allicance for Consumer Education. *Inhalant Abuse Prevention: a facilitator's guide.* Washington, DC: Alliance for Consumer Education; 2006. Available at: www.uproarorg.org/resources/ace_facilitators_guide.pdf

35 Cairney S, Maruff P, Burns C, *et al.* The neurobehavioural consequences of petrol (gasoline) sniffing. *Neurosci Biobehav Rev.* 2002; **26**(1): 81–90.

36 Yücel M, Takagi M, Walterfang M, *et al.* Toulene misuse and long-term harms: a systematic review of the neuropsychological and neuroimaging literature. *Neurosci Biobehav Rev.* 2008; **32**(5): 910–26.

37 Campbell A. *Experiences of and Attitudes to Head Shop Psychoactive Substances among Adolescents* [dissertation]. Dublin: Trinity College Dublin; 2011.

38 Kelleher C, Christie R, Lalor K, *et al. An Overview of New Psychoactive Substances and the Outlets Supplying Them.* Dublin: National Advisory Committee on Drugs; 2011.

39 Long J. Conference on psychoactive drugs sold in head shops and online. *Drugnet Ireland.* 2010; **33**: 1–3.

40 Van Hout MC, Brennan R. Plant food for thought: a qualitative study of mephedrone use in Ireland. *Drug-Educ Prev Polic.* 2010; **18**(5): 371–81.

41 O'Reilly F, McAuliffe R, Long J. Users experiences of cathinones sold in head shops and online. *Irish J Psychol Med.* 2011; **28**(1): S4–7.

42 Wood DM, Greene SL, Dargan PI. Clinical pattern of toxicity associated with the novel synthetic cathinone mephedrone. *Emerg Med J.* 2011; **28**(4): 280–2.

43 Wilkins C, Sweetsur P. Differences in harm from legal BZP/TFMPP party pills between North Island and South Island users in New Zealand: a case of effective industry self-regulation? *Int J Drug Policy.* 2010; **21**(1): 86–90.

CHAPTER 4

Why do we worry about teenage substance use?

INTRODUCTION

There is a complex relationship between substance use and adolescent development. The use of alcohol and other substances are seen within some cultures as a rite of passage or the start of adulthood. It is important that staff working with substance using adolescents have a good understanding of the potential adverse consequences. Many teenagers will argue that their substance use has not caused any problems. They may assert that adults need to calm down about the risks. In this chapter we outline the range of risks and problems potentially associated with substance use in adolescence. This should facilitate you in having an informed and balanced discussion with teenagers about the potential hazards of their substance use.

ACCIDENTS HAPPEN . . .

One of the reasons people choose to consume alcohol and other drugs is that they cause us to drop our inhibitions and relax. While relaxing is good, it really means that we care less about what we are doing and what is occurring around us. We can lose ourselves in the moment and dwell less on the future. This can all be very pleasant. One of the problems with this substance-induced effect is that it can also cause us to take risks. We are more impulsive. We avoid considering how things might go wrong and ignore the longer-term potential negative consequences. Therefore, we can behave out of character and do things we wouldn't normally do. While this may lead to some genuine fun and innocent silliness, it can get us into trouble. This trouble usually results in nothing more than some social embarrassment the next day as we are reminded of things we did and said. On other occasions it can be more serious. Our behaviour may have put our health, or that of others, under threat or caused real harm. It may have seriously damaged a relationship with friends, work colleagues, family or partner. Although intoxication is usually accompanied by improved mood, it is unpredictable and it can contribute to negative feelings. The latter can lead to aggressive and antisocial behaviour, which can again damage relationships or bring us into contact with the police.

While these issues are features of intoxication in general across the age span, in adolescents the intoxication effects, both good and bad, are exaggerated. Again remember that teenagers are *apprentice adults* (*see* Chapter 2). They are still *learning* how to problem-solve, how to socialise and how to manage their own emotions. As discussed in Chapter 2, they already have a mismatch between their drive towards fun and their ability to restrain themselves where there is potential for risk. Their brain is structured such that the engine or accelerator is a little more powerful than the brakes. As Aristotle noted, they 'are heated by nature as drunken men by wine'. Unfortunately, the impact of any intoxicant is to further exaggerate the mismatch between the accelerator and the braking system in the brain. To paraphrase Aristotle, they end up heated by nature *and* by wine, or vodka, or cocaine. When this reality is considered alongside their lack of life experience, it is easy to see how accidents happen.

The adolescent years are generally a time of excellent physical health. Where deaths occur among young males aged 12–25 years, there are two dominant contributors. Accidents account for about one-third of deaths. These include deaths in falls, road traffic collisions, fires and drowning. Alcohol is involved in about one-third of these deaths.[1,2] There are also occasional deaths from acute alcohol or drug intoxication (i.e. accidental overdoses) and some deaths occur via intoxication-fuelled assaults. Another one-third of deaths in young males, especially in older teenagers and young adults, are due to suicide. While patterns vary across the globe, somewhere between one- and two-thirds of these young men are intoxicated when they take their own lives, typically in very impulsive acts.[1,2]

While deaths grab the headlines, there are also many teenagers seriously injured in accidents linked to their own or their peers' intoxication. Indeed, the public health community has argued that these injuries are such predictable consequences of risky behaviour that we should not use expressions such as 'road traffic accidents'. The word 'accident' suggests that it is some random, unforeseen event, out of human control. This is rarely the case. It is suggested that the word 'collision' is used. If we view and discuss such deaths as accidents, there is a danger that society won't learn from the error made by the person who was injured or died. While media and society often highlight the role of drugs in deaths, there is commonly a reluctance to highlight the role that alcohol plays in these events.[3]

In addition to deaths and injuries linked to the disinhibiting effects of intoxication, unplanned pregnancy and sexual health problems can also occur. Teenagers commonly report unplanned sexual encounters while intoxicated (*see* Chapter 14). This can lead to sexually transmitted infections, some of which can have long-term implications for fertility and health.

IMPACT OF DRUG AND ALCOHOL USE ON THE DEVELOPING BRAIN

There is a growing body of research that indicates that early exposure by teenagers to drug or alcohol abuse tends to disrupt the normal development of the brain outlined in Chapter 2. In other words, regular exposure to these substances during the early- or mid-teenage years tends to change the teenage brain. This evidence has emerged from a number of studies conducted on young people who are abusing alcohol and drugs, using technologies such as magnetic resonance imaging. As outlined in Chapter 2, neuronal connections are established and pruned, depending on their use or otherwise during adolescence. The presence of potent neuro-stimulator substances, whether alcohol or drugs, appear to influence the process of neuronal connections thereby altering brain function and structure.[4]

The biological changes induced by regular alcohol abuse during adolescence may also explain something that has been observed many decades ago by scientists and those treating addiction. It is a fact that the earlier in life alcohol abuse commences, the greater the risk of dependence in adulthood and also the harder it is to treat that alcohol dependence in adulthood.[5] Regular heavy drinking during this phase of brain development may cause enduring changes, leaving these young people vulnerable to a latter, more severe alcohol dependence in adulthood.[4]

In 2007, the surgeon general in the United States published a report outlining the need to urgently reduce the level of alcohol abuse among American teenagers.[6] He was prompted to do this because of

> new, disturbing research which indicates that the developing adolescent brain may be particularly susceptible to long-term negative consequences from alcohol use . . . alcohol consumption has the potential to trigger long-term biological changes that may have detrimental effects on the developing adolescent brain.[6]

More recently, a review of the literature commented,

> studies have reported altered brain structure and function in alcohol dependent

or abusing adolescents . . . with smaller frontal & hippocampal volumes . . . suggesting that early adolescence may be a period of heightened risk to alcohol's neurotoxic effects.[4]

There is also a growing literature that demonstrates the negative impact drugs other than alcohol have on brain structure and functioning.[7,8]

INCREASED RISK OF ADDICTION AND PROGRESSION TO MORE DANGEROUS DRUGS

Modern theories of addiction now view it as a problem with a neurobiological basis. Nora Volkow, Director of the US National Institute on Drug Abuse, has called addiction 'a pathology of motivation and choice'.[9] Based on the findings from brain scan research and observations of patterns of substance abuse over decades, Volkow and others believe that people who have become addicted to drugs have damaged their ability to make healthy choices. Their past substance use has caused changes to their limbic system that result in increased drive to engage in drug use. Past exposure to prolonged substance use has also damaged their ability to suppress such cravings, via impairment in certain functions of their frontal lobes. You will recall from Chapter 2 that the limbic system is analogous to an engine or accelerator in a car, while the frontal lobe acts like the brake. This modern theory of addiction states that chronic drug use increases the 'engine' activity while simultaneously damaging the 'braking' mechanism.[10] The bottom line is that these brain changes make it difficult for substance users to stop using and leave them vulnerable to relapse if they do manage to stop.

ALCOHOL MAY BE THE MAIN 'GATEWAY' DRUG

The vast majority of drug abusing teenagers we encounter in our clinical work have progressed to drug use following a period of alcohol abuse. A substantial body of international research seems to support this observation.[11] Drunkenness appears to act as a stepping stone to illicit drug use. For example, we have found that 80% of teenagers who have used cocaine were drunk when they first took it. Inhibitions are dropped while drunk. The line of cocaine is harder to resist.

If teenagers are used to getting drunk on all social occasions while out with their peers from the ages of 13 or 14 years, it appears that some will find things boring by the time they reach 16 years. Getting drunk is no longer enough. Some of these 16-year-olds, after their couple of years of binge drinking, decide to seek other substances for a new 'buzz'. In most Western countries, they now have access to a broad range of cheap drugs.

Apart from concerns about risk of progressing to abuse of other drugs, early-onset drinking increases the likelihood that a young person will develop alcohol dependence as an adult. It has been observed that alcohol-dependent adults who commenced regular drinking prior to the age of 15 years have poorer outcomes and more relapses.[5]

In a nutshell, during the period of brain development in the teenage years, the brain is somewhat plastic and additional changes can occur as a result of repeatedly bathing the brain in potent neurostimulatory substances via regular substance use. These changes can endure into adulthood and may become permanent.

CANNABIS AND SCHIZOPHRENIA

These changes to brain development may explain the observed increased risk of schizophrenia among those with a history of regular cannabis use during the mid-teenage years. The growing consensus among the scientific community is that regular cannabis use during mid-adolescence doubles the risk of developing schizophrenia-type illnesses in adulthood.[12] The hypothesis to explain this observation is that some teenagers experience a change in the dopamine neural networks within their brain that is caused by their regular cannabis use. These induced changes leave them vulnerable to developing schizophrenia in the future.

It is probable that some teenagers are more susceptible to the negative effects of cannabis than others and there is research to suggest that this vulnerability may be genetic in origin.[13] In other words, teenagers with certain genes may actually be able to smoke cannabis without great risk to their mental health, while others may be at high risk arising from their cannabis use.

There are analogous phenomena in other areas of healthcare. They are known as *gene–environment interactions*. For example, we know that sun exposure increases the risk of development of skin cancers such as melanoma. We also know that certain skin types, determined genetically, are particularly vulnerable to the risks of sun exposure. Those of us with very pale complexions are more vulnerable than people with darker skin types. People with freckly, pale skin that is prone to sunburn can take precautions by applying sunblock in order to manage this risk or, alternatively, they can avoid exposing their skin to the midday sun. Unfortunately, the factors that make some teenagers vulnerable to this risk of schizophrenia following cannabis use are not so obvious. While we can quickly look at our child's skin type to appraise the potential risk from sun exposure, there is no current method for knowing if we do or do not have the sort of brain that is vulnerable to the schizophrenia-inducing effects of cannabis smoking.

When making this point about the increased risk of schizophrenia and cannabis use it is important to give teenagers a measured, proportionate but accurate message. In reality about 1% of 'ordinary' 15-year-olds will go on to develop schizophrenia in adulthood. If one followed up a group of 15-year-olds who are regular cannabis users for the same period of time, one would find that 2% or 3% will develop schizophrenia.[12] The flip side of this is that 97%–98% of regular cannabis smokers will *not* develop schizophrenia. Hence, it is important not to scaremonger teenagers by exagerating the link between cannabis and schizophrenia. However, it is equally important that they are informed that it will increase their risk of developing this most devastating of mental illnesses by a small but definite amount.

The fact that the absolute risk is low does not mean that parents can be complacent. If our children get sunburned, this increases the risk of skin cancer later in life. Despite the reality that the vast majority of children who get sunburned will not get skin cancer, this doesn't stop us taking active efforts to ensure that our children wear sunblock when they go out in the sunshine. We do what we can to protect our children from serious dangers.

IMPACT OF CANNABIS ON MEMORY AND MOTIVATION

There is growing evidence that cannabis use has a negative impact on cognitive functioning. In 2012, results were published from the Dunedin study, a long-term follow-up of people born in a New Zealand city in the early 1970s.[14] The study found that people who abused cannabis during their mid-teenage years demonstrated a decline in their IQ, or intelligence, when followed up at the age of 38 years. In fact, they found that group demonstrated a 9-point fall in IQ, on average. Those who started abusing cannabis in their early twenties didn't demonstrate the same IQ drop but those who started as teenagers did. This again points to the fact that the brain is particularly susceptible to the negative impacts of substances during adolescence. Hence, the public health message should be: 'If you're going to smoke cannabis, leave it until you're into your twenties'.

The Dunedin study is not alone in indicating a negative impact of cannabis on cognitive functioning. There is substantial research that indicates that aspects of memory are impaired in adults who smoke cannabis heavily.[15] Cannabis users appear to recognise these negative effects of their drug use themselves. Adam Winstock, founder of the Global Drugs Survey, has conducted web-based interviews with cannabis users. The two main health worries among users related to the negative impact that cannabis has both on their mental health and on their memory.

PHYSICAL HEALTH IMPACTS OF ADOLESCENTS SUBSTANCE USE

Heavy and regular use of alcohol by large numbers of adolescents has resulted in a growing number of cases of cirrhosis in young adults in their late twenties and early thirties. Girls are now drinking as much as, if not more than, boys. Females appear more vulnerable to the liver-damaging effects of alcohol use. While cirrhosis at the age of 30 may seem like a catastrophic outcome, this possibility may generate little concern for a 14-year-old, for whom 30-year-olds are 'ancient'. Heavy episodic drinking is also a contributor to acute pancreatitis. This is now seen with increasing frequency in older teenagers and young adults. Alcohol is also a very significant contributor to adult-onset epilepsy.

Stimulant drugs speed up the heart rate. This can lead to arrhythmias, which can cause sudden death. Cocaine has been associated with myocardial infarcts, or 'heart attacks' in young adults. Alcohol can very occasionally cause major damage to the heart muscle via a cardiomyopathy. Although temporary, this can be fatal, given the importance of the heart for maintaining life.

A small minority of adolescents opt to inject drugs such as heroin and cocaine. Drug injection is associated with greatly increased risk of accidental overdose. It is also linked with risk of complicated wounds called abscesses and, more seriously, an infection of the valves in the heart (endocarditis). Sharing of injecting equipment can result in the spread of viral infections such as HIV, hepatitis C and hepatitis B.

If a teenage girl is abusing substances while pregnant, damage can be done to the developing foetus. As outlined earlier in this chapter, and in Chapter 14, unplanned sex is a frequent feature of substance abuse. Many girls do not realise they are pregnant until 2 or 3 months have passed. They may continue to abuse substances during this time. Unfortunately, the foetus is most vulnerable to the teratogenic effects of substances during these early months. Perhaps the most dangerous drug to the foetus is alcohol. Many children are born each year with foetal alcohol syndrome, or foetal alcohol spectrum disorder.[16] Core psychological features of foetal alcohol syndrome include learning difficulties, impulsivity and overactivity.

POTENTIAL MENTAL HEALTH IMPACTS OF ADOLESCENT SUBSTANCE USE

Mental health can be adversely affected by substance abuse. Earlier we have outlined the evidence that adolescent cannabis use can increase the risk of schizophrenia later in life. It is also clear that cannabis use, and abuse of stimulant drugs, contributes to much poorer outcomes in teenagers with illnesses such as schizophrenia and bipolar disorder, even if drugs had no role in causing the condition.

The novel psychoactive substances, sometimes called 'legal highs' or 'head shop drugs', also seem to have a particular propensity to cause acute deteriorations in mental health in those with and without an underlying mental health condition. In light of the facts that these drugs have much in common with cannabis and stimulant drugs, this is not a surprise.

Heavy regular use of any drug is very commonly associated with low mood and increased anxiety symptoms. These symptoms can mimic many psychiatric disorders. This makes it difficult for psychiatrists to assess people who are using drugs regularly. When teenagers reduce or cease their substance use, they generally experience an improvement in any coexisting mental health symptoms.

The complex interaction between symptoms of mental illness and substance abuse is most evident when considering psychotic symptoms. Psychotic symptoms include hearing voices and delusions (*see* Chapter 13). Delusions are fixed, false beliefs that seem utterly real to the person. They are frequently paranoid in content – for example, the person believing that they are being spied upon or poisoned. Table 4.1 outlines the potential linkages between such symptoms and substance abuse. Staff assessing a psychotic teenager who is abusing substances will need to give consideration to the type of substance, the intensity of recent use and the timing of last use when undertaking their assessment. However, this information may not be available if the teenager is acutely distressed or intoxicated. Table 4.2 outlines the range of negative mental health symptoms and problems that can occur in the context of substance use and abuse.

As discussed earlier, substance abuse plays a major role in suicides among young people.[1] In one study of youth suicide in Ireland, it was observed that 58% were very intoxicated (blood alcohol concentration >160 mg%) at the time of their death.[2] Substance abuse can lead to an ongoing deterioration in mood. It can also negatively impact relationships. Against this backdrop, acute intoxication can generate a further dip in mood, contribute to the row, which causes immediate upset and increases impulsivity to the extent that people decide to kill themselves. Consequently, it is not a surprise that many deaths among adolescents with substance use problems are suicides.

IMPACT OF SUBSTANCE USE ON SOCIAL DEVELOPMENT
Lack of effective coping skills

Research into human development tells us that there are often crucial and brief windows of opportunity for acquisition of certain skills. For example, looking at the development of language, research has been conducted on that small number of youngsters who have grown up in environments where they have not been exposed to any language, usually because of extreme neglect and abuse. These unfortunate children fail to develop normal language ever, no matter how much tuition or exposure they have to language in later childhood. Noam Chomsky[17] has hypothesised that there is what he called the 'language acquisition device'. This 'switches on' in our brain during the first year of our life to tune us into language and it equips us to learn language rapidly and effectively. However, there seems to be a crucial window during which we can

TABLE 4.1 Substance abuse and psychotic presentations: 'drug-induced psychosis'

Type of psychotic presentation	Substances potentially associated
Intoxication mimicking psychosis	Stimulants, cannabis, ecstasy, LSD, solvents, NPSs
Brief psychotic reactions	Stimulants, cannabis, NPSs
Flashbacks	LSD, cannabis, ecstasy, NPSs
Drug-induced relapse	Stimulants, cannabis, NPSs
Withdrawal states	Barbiturates, benzodiazepines, alcohol, GBH

Note: NPSs, novel psychoactive substances (e.g mephadrone)

TABLE 4.2 Mental health symptoms and time lapsed after last substance use

Intoxication symptoms	Disinhibition
	Blackouts
	Anxiety and/or panic
	Compulsion to use more
	Delusions and paranoia
	Hallucinations
	Aggression
	Confusion
	Unpredictable mood change
Symptoms on Days 1–7	Crash in mood – intense hopelessness
	Ongoing anxiety/panic
	Irritability
	Poor self-care
	Delusions and paranoia induced by withdrawals
	Hallucinations
	Confusion precipitated by withdrawals
Symptoms on Week 2+	Drug-induced depressive episode
	Drug-induced manic episode
	Drug-induced anxiety disorder
	Drug-induced psychosis

acquire this skill and those youngsters who were devoid of human contact and the opportunity to learn language during those first few years of life find themselves struggling to learn it subsequently. They have missed their window of opportunity.

During adolescence we acquire a broad repertoire of problem-solving styles and coping strategies. This equips us to deal with the 'slings and arrows of life'. If an adolescent boy copes with all of life's difficulties by using substances to blank out problems or deal with unpleasant emotions, he inevitably misses out on the huge learning opportunity that the teenage years provide. He fails to acquire other more effective coping strategies. He can consequently arrive into adulthood with this single strategy, resorting to intoxication, every time life gets difficult. That subset of teenagers, who turn to substance or alcohol misuse as a coping strategy, are a particularly at-risk and damaged group. These children may have missed their window of opportunity to acquire adaptive social and other skills. This may leave them compromised in terms of their future ability to acquire and develop healthier and effective coping strategies and social interactional styles, even if they do subsequently cease use of drugs or alcohol in adulthood.

Fun without drink?

Across all cultures, young children aged 4–10 years have fun without any real difficulty. They have a great ability to enjoy themselves when surrounded by other young children. They do this without alcohol or other intoxicants. It appears that many people in countries such as Ireland, Britain, Australia and New Zealand seem to lose this ability as they head towards adulthood. A growing majority of us appear to believe that it would be impossible to have a laugh without alcohol, even in the company of our nearest and dearest.

If this is true, something must happen to those of us from Anglo-Saxon cultures between the ages of 8 and 28 years that causes us to lose our ability to have fun in the company of our friends, peers and family without intoxication. In contrast, adults from most other cultures, especially Mediterranean and Asian countries, appear to retain this ability. In our Anglo-Saxon cultures, do we choose to get drunk to recreate the disinhibited freedom of our childhoods, or could it be that our routine use of intoxication in almost all social and celebratory settings from mid-adolescence onwards causes us to permanently lose this ability, setting in motion a vicious circle?

If children are to have any chance of being able to enjoy themselves, enjoy the company of peers without the crutch of alcohol as adults, then we argue that our societies should strive to delay their drinking for as long as possible. Indeed, this is one of the main reasons why we should delay children's drinking. If they, at the age of 14, 15 or 16 years, find it necessary to get drunk, or intoxicated on drugs, to enjoy a night out with their friends or peers there is little hope that they will ever as adults be able to enjoy social events and settings without substance use. However, if they manage to make it to the age of 17, 18 or 19 years without routinely getting drunk in social situations they will probably be able to enjoy themselves and interact with peers in a fun, relaxed manner without the artificial assistance of alcohol or other intoxicants. Later, as young adults, they may of course decide to supplement the social night out with the addition of alcohol, and may even get drunk the odd time. The difference is that they won't *need* to drink to socialise.

If adults in our societies accept the notion that 15- and 16-year-olds need to have alcohol to enjoy their social life, we are really communicating to them a dreadfully nihilistic and hopeless message about their capacity to have fun and feel joy in the company of their peers. Hello Sunday Morning (http://hellosundaymorning.org) is an online, international organisation that seeks to constructively challenge the link between alcohol and fun.

Other adverse social impacts of substance use

Adolescents who use substances frequently perform less well at school. Substance use, due to acute intoxication, withdrawal and possible neurobiological effects can affect memory and concentration, making it more difficult to learn in school. Some of these effects may also make it more likely that the teenager ends up breaking school rules. Educational outcomes are therefore poorer on average.

Substance use has the potential to damage relationships with parents. This may be a consequence of the irritability and anger associated with substance use and may arise out of conflict between adolescent and parent over his or her choice to use substances. A parent's trust in their teenager can be poor after it emerges that the adolescent is using drugs. Where trust has been damaged, adolescents tend to underestimate the amount of time and effort it takes to rebuild it.

As adolescents become more involved in substance use, their peer network tends to change. They spend increasing time with other substance-using teenagers and can lose contact with non-substance-using friends. It can then be difficult to re-establish these friendships if they later cease substance use. They may end up being identified by the wider peer network as 'a stoner', 'a junkie' or 'a drunkard'. If so, they will find themselves increasingly excluded by the 'ordinary' non-substance-using peer group. This represents yet another example of a vicious circle, which can perpetuate a teenager's journey into more problematic substance use.

Drugs and alcohol can be expensive. Teenagers can rapidly find themselves in debt, especially if they use potent short-acting drugs such as cocaine, amphetamines or heroin. Drug markets change very quickly. In Ireland in 2012, there were increasing reports of significant debts associated with cannabis use. Some Irish teenagers report spending up to €50 a day on cannabis. This was unheard of 5 years earlier. This has occurred against the backdrop of a move away from cannabis resin towards herbal cannabis and a substantial increase in potency. The costs associated with drug use cause some teenagers to choose to engage in criminal activity to fund their use, so called acquisitive crime. Intoxication can be associated with criminal activity ranging from public disorder to an alcohol- or drug-fuelled homicide. This activity generates criminal charges and increases the pace of social marginalisation.

Adolescents in the modern world live public lives and engage much wider networks of friends and acquaintances than previous generations. They achieve this via active participation in social media (e.g. Facebook, Twitter). This brings some potential benefits for adolescents in the twenty-first century. It also creates new challenges and can cause real problems in the context of substance abuse. A relatively minor 'mistake' made while intoxicated can become widely known by peers very quickly. Having sex or getting into a row with the wrong person can result in being rapidly tagged as 'a slapper' or 'a psycho'. If it becomes known that a teenager is abusing a substance, possibly because of comments made by the teenager him- or herself on his or her Facebook page, this can quickly snowball.

Few drugs have been more widely studied than cannabis in long-term research projects. The focus on cannabis is largely down to the fact that it is the most widely used illicit drug in adolescence. It is therefore relatively easy to study. The consequences of using amphetamines, cocaine, benzodiazepines and the new drugs like mephedrone are likely to be as bad, if not worse. When the social outcomes of adolescent cannabis users have been reviewed it is observed that they are much more likely to function poorly as adults when compared to adolescents who don't use drugs. They have poorer educational attainment, lower mood, more marital breakdown, greater criminal convictions and poorer employment history. After reviewing the scientific literature in 2007, Patton, *et al.*[18] concluded quite starkly, 'cannabis was the drug of choice for life's future losers'.

CONCLUSION

Substance use at any age carries risks, but many of these risks are greater during adolescence. They exacerbate adolescents' pre-existing tendency towards impulsivity. This can result in accidents and behaviour, which causes harm to self or others. While physical health consequences of substance use typically do not become apparent until adulthood, mental health problems increase in adolescents who abuse substances. Alcohol and drug use are also associated with suicidal behaviour, via unpredictable impact on mood, impaired problem-solving and increased impulsivity. There is growing evidence that the adolescent brain seems particularly vulnerable to the neurotoxic effects of substances. This may explain the impaired cognitive functioning demonstrated by people who begin using at a young age. Early-onset use is associated with greater risk of dependence in adulthood. Regular use of substances during adolescence can result in teenagers failing to develop other adaptive coping strategies and may result in them becoming reliant upon intoxication as the central strategy to socialise. Substance abuse during adolescence is also associated with poorer functioning in a range of social domains such as school and family. It also increases the likelihood of criminal justice problems.

KEY POINTS

- The brain is developing and changing during adolescence. Consequently, it may be particularly vulnerable to the apparent ability of substances to induce enduring and negative changes to brain structure and functioning.
- Disinhibition associated with intoxication contributes to accidents and other risk behaviour.
- There is a strong relationship between suicide and substance use, especially in older adolescent males.
- In cultures that are accepting of drunkenness, alcohol may be the main 'gateway' or 'stepping stone' drug, as it provides young people with their first experience of intoxication.
- While adolescents often report that substances help them to socialise, by taking away their inhibitions and anxieties, its longer-term effect may be to hinder their social development. They may come to rely on intoxication in order to socialise.

FURTHER READING

- European Monitoring Centre for Drugs and Drug Addiction (EMCDDA). *Addiction Neurobiology: ethical and social implications.* Lisbon: EMCDDA; 2009. Available at: www.emcdda.europa.eu/publications/monographs/neurobiology (in language that is easily accessible, the report presents the complex brain processes involved in addiction and the ethical implications inherent to current addiction research).
- US National Institute on Drug Abuse – teaching packets on addiction. Available at: www.drugabuse.gov/publications/term/210/TeachingPackets
- Global Drugs Survey. Gathers information on international drug use trends using data gathered directly from drug users. http://globaldrugsurvey.com/

➡ US National Institute on Alcohol Abuse and Alcoholism. *Adolescent Development and Alcohol Use.* Available at: https://webmeeting.nih.gov/p95927495/ (web-based presentation with audio, summarising aspects of adolescent development and harms associated with teenage drinking – 25 minutes long).

REFERENCES

1 Allebeck P, Allgulander C, Henningsohn L, *et al.* Causes of death in a cohort of 50 465 young men: validity of recorded suicide as underlying cause of death. *Scand J Soc Med.* 1991; **19**(4): 242–7.

2 Bedford D, O'Farrell A, Howell F. Blood alcohol levels in persons who died from accidents and suicide. *Ir Med J.* 2006; **99**(3): 80–3.

3 Slater MD, Long M, Ford VL. Alcohol, illegal drugs, violent crime, and traffic-related and other unintended injuries in U.S. local and national news. *J Stud Alcohol.* 2006; **67**(6): 904–10.

4 Casey BJ, Jones RM. Neurobiology of the adolescent brain and behavior: implications for substance use disorders. *J Am Acad Child Adolesc Psychiatry.* 2010: **49**(12): 1189–201.

5 Hingson RW, Heeren T, Winter MR. Age at drinking onset and alcohol dependence: age at onset, duration, and severity. *Arch Paediatr Adolesc Med.* 2006; **160**(7): 739–46.

6 Office of the Surgeon General. *The Surgeon General's Call to Action to Prevent and Reduce Underage Drinking: a guide to action for families.* Rockville, MD: US Department of Health and Human Services; 2007.

7 Demirakca T, Sartorius A, Ende G, *et al.* Diminished gray matter in the hippocampus of cannabis users: possible protective effects of cannabidiol. *Drug Alcohol Depend.* 2011; **114**(2): 242–5.

8 Urban NB, Girgis RR, Talbot PS, *et al.* Sustained recreational use of Ecstasy is associated with altered pre and postsynaptic markers of serotonin transmission in neocortical areas: a PET study with [11C]DASB and [11C]MDL 100907. *Neuropsychopharmacology.* 2012; **37**(6): 1465–73.

9 Kalivas PW, Volkow ND. The neural basis of addiction: a pathology of motivation and choice. *Am J Psychiatry.* 2005: **162**(8): 1403–13.

10 Carter A, Capps B, Hall W. *Addiction Neurobiology: ethical and social implications.* Lisbon: European Monitoring Centre for Drugs and Drug Addiction; 2009.

11 Fergusson DM, Boden JM, Horwood LJ. The developmental antecedents of illicit drug use: evidence from a 25-year longitudinal study. *Drug Alcohol Depend.* 2008; **96**(1–2): 165–77.

12 Arseneault L, Cannon M, Witton J, *et al.* Causal association between cannabis and psychosis: examination of the evidence. *Br J Psychiatry.* 2004; **184**(2): 110–17.

13 Caspi A, Moffitt TE, Cannon M, *et al.* Moderation of the effect of adolescent-onset cannabis use on adult psychosis by a functional polymorphism in the catechol-O-methyltransferase gene: longitudinal evidence of a gene X environment interaction. *Biol Psychiatry.* 2005; **57**(10): 1117–27.

14 Meier MH, Caspi A, Ambler A, *et al.* Persistent cannabis users show neuropsychological decline from childhood to midlife. *Proc Natl Acad Sci U S A.* 2012; **109**(40): 2657–64.

15 Solowij N, Battisti R. The chronic effects of cannabis on memory in humans: a review. *Curr Drug Abuse Rev.* 2008; **1**(1): 81–98.

16 Mattson SN, Riley EP. A review of the neurobehavioral deficits in children with fetal alcohol syndrome or prenatal exposure to alcohol. *Alcohol Clin Exp Res.* 2006; **22**(2): 279–94.

17 Chomsky N. Recent contributions to the theory of innate ideas. *Synthese.* 1967; **17**(1): 2–11.

18 Patton GC, Coffey C, Lynskey MT, *et al.* Trajectories of adolescent alcohol and cannabis use into young adulthood. *Addiction.* 2007; **102**(4): 607–15.

CHAPTER 5

Why do some teenagers abuse substances? Risk and protective factors

In previous chapters we presented the idea that teenagers can be considered 'apprentice adults'. During adolescence, their task is to pick up the social skills to equip them for adulthood. Like any group of apprentices some will do better than others. Teenagers vary a great deal in the pace at which they master the skills necessary for adulthood. Some teenagers arrive into adolescence with highly developed skills and then rapidly and easily add to these. Others are less fortunate and may enter adolescence with poorer than average ability to manage frustration or have limited communication abilities, for example. The mentoring that a teenager receives during their adolescence, from parents, teachers and other important adults in their lives will also have a bearing on the ease with which they move through their teenage years. Lastly, the environment they find themselves learning within will clearly influence their skills development.

Researchers have identified a myriad of factors that increase the risk that adolescents run into problems during their teenage years. Experimentation with drugs and alcohol and the subsequent development of significant problems around these substances represent one of many potential hazards that teenagers encounter.

Historically, research has focused on risk factors, seeking to identify the individual, family, peer, school and community characteristics associated with *increased* risk of developing problems such as substance use. More recently, there have been efforts to understand the variability in outcomes among teenagers by focusing on *resilience* or *protective* factors. This strengths-based approach facilitates a more positive dialogue with both teenagers and families.

It causes those who work with such teenagers to identify their pre-existing talents and positive protective factors.

Interestingly, many factors that reduce the likelihood of a teenager developing a substance use problem are also factors that protect against a range of other undesirable outcomes for teenagers. The presence of these *general protective factors* also reduces the risk of deliberate self-harm, sexual risk behaviour, aggression and emotional problems.

GENERAL PROTECTIVE FACTORS: THE 40 DEVELOPMENTAL ASSETS

While many researchers and scientific review papers have sought to compile lists of protective factors, the Search Institute in the United States has put together a very useful list of 40 protective factors. They view protective factors as *assets* that a young person can have in their lives. They are the '40 Developmental Assets'. (The full list can be quickly accessed via an Internet search of that term.)

There are 20 *internal assets*. These are features of individual teenagers, each representing a potential, intrinsic, psychological characteristic of the person. While parents and schools can nurture internal assets, they cannot be put in place externally if the teenager has not developed them. There are also 20 *external assets* related to supports that exist around the teenager. They are provided by family, school and community. Developmental psychologists talk about the idea of 'scaffolding' around teenagers. They conceptualise teenagers as rising but somewhat unstable buildings that need a range of external supports to ensure they stay up and to permit additional height to be put on the building. These external assets provide that scaffolding.

Research indicates that adolescents fortunate to have 30 or more development assets are at greatly reduced risk of many negative outcomes during their adolescent years (*see* Figure 5.1).[1] They exhibit lower rates of substance use, less-frequent aggression and violence and lower rates of self-harm and depression. In contrast, young people who have fewer than 10 of the developmental assets exhibit high rates of these same problems. As with all protective factors, their presence does not *guarantee* good outcomes and nor does their absence make a bad outcome inevitable. Each additional asset simply increases the likelihood that teenagers will avoid problem behaviours.

The attraction of the 40 Developmental Assets model is its simplicity. It is easy to explain to teenagers, families and professionals. Because of its focus on strengths, it facilitates positive conversation. Perhaps its only weakness is a consequence of its simplicity – each asset is given equal weight. However, research on outcomes in adolescents indicates that some of these assets confer greater protection than others.[2]

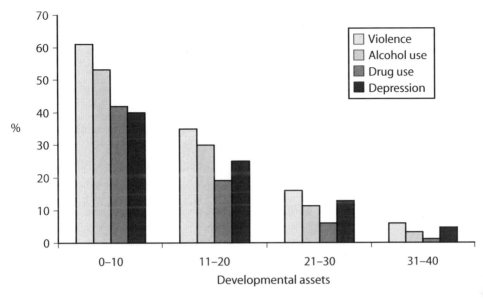

FIGURE 5.1 Developmental assets and coexisting problems in teenagers[1]

Internal assets

Many studies have highlighted the importance of a *commitment to learning* and education among young people.[2] The first five internal assets (assets 21–25) capture this commitment to learning. Adolescents who are invested in their education and report a positive connection to school are at an advantage. Those who have developed a habit of doing their homework each evening are also at an advantage.

Teenagers who have a range of *positive values* demonstrate reduced risk of substance use problems. Internal assets 26–31 focus on these positive values. Adolescents who are outward looking, demonstrating care for others and who believe that the world should be fair tend to be less likely to drift into substance use. Those who believe in the importance of integrity, of being honest themselves and who accept personal responsibility for their own behaviours are also at a reduced risk of negative outcomes.

For obvious reasons, young people who exhibit restraint are at reduced risk of substance use. This protection has its origins in their belief that just because something is fun does not mean that it should be done. Restraint is a characteristic that has been shown to be enduring over time and protective through adolescence into adulthood via some interesting and simple experiments. Famously, in the 1960s, Walter Mischel of Stanford University conducted the *marshmallow test* with young children.[3] In this test the child was told they could have a marshmallow immediately, or they could have two if they waited for 15 minutes while the adult left the room. Children who resisted the temptation to eat the marshmallow were viewed to have exhibited restraint or *deferred gratification*. When these children were followed up through adolescence and adulthood they had better outcomes across many aspects of social functioning, including lower rates of substance abuse.

Internal assets 32–36 relate to *social competencies*. It is not surprising that those youth who demonstrated greater natural ability in areas of social competence also encounter less difficulty on their journey through adolescence. Young people who have better cognitive skills, are more organised and have greater ability to problem solve and plan, demonstrate lower rates of substance use. Having good interpersonal skills is also beneficial. Teenagers who can stand on their own two feet and not be swept along by the behaviours of peers also have an advantage.

The last group of internal assets relate to a *positive sense of identity*. Adolescents who understand that they have an influence over their own life exhibit lower rates of risk behaviour. In the 1950s, Julian Rotter[4] wrote about locus of control. It is better to a have an internal locus of control, as opposed to an external locus of control. Teenagers who perceive themselves as powerless over their own lives and futures are more likely to be drawn to short-term pleasures.

It is good for teenagers to feel that their life has a purpose. It is also beneficial in terms of general mental health outcomes for adolescents to be relatively optimistic about their future.

Having high self-esteem is another developmental asset. The impact of self-esteem on risk-taking behaviour is interesting. There is much research that indicates that teenagers with higher self-esteem are *more* likely to experiment with substances.[5] The observation is counter-intuitive but appears to relate to the view that those with high self-esteem may have an inflated sense of their ability to manage challenging situations. Some teenagers with high self-esteem will exhibit the type of confidence–competence mismatch described in Chapter 2. Many of us who work in adolescent substance abuse services will notice that teenagers who run into significant difficulty around drug or alcohol abuse exhibit low self-esteem. Among the group of adolescents who experiment with substances, it is those with lower self-esteem who appear more likely to develop a substance use disorder.

External assets

The Search Institute cites 20 external assets. The first six relate to the quality of the *supportive environment* around the teenager to facilitate their social learning. The quality of the relationships with mentors is an important influence on the pace at which people will learn. Family is important. Teenagers who say they live in families with high levels of support exhibit lower rates of substance use. Young people who can talk to at least one of their parents in a positive manner and indicate that they are willing to go to this parent with problems they encounter are at an advantage. It is also important that teenagers have other adults that they can turn to for advice. These adults might include grandparents, teachers, coaches etc. These adults can have a particularly important role where the young person is experiencing problems *with* parents. Other aspects of the environment around the teenager are also important. These include caring neighbours and going to a school that they perceive as providing encouragement.

External assets 7–10 highlight the importance of how community and society views and treats teenagers. These assets throw down a challenge to Western society because they ask us to *view adolescents positively*. We are encouraged to regard teenagers as a resource. In light of our tendency to have a negative stereotypical view of teenagers, it is possible that many teenagers grow up without these assets. Teenagers who say young people are given roles within their community are at an advantage even if they, as individual teenagers, choose not to take on such roles. The very fact that the community is willing to give responsibility to teenagers seems protective in and of itself. However, an additional layer of protection is provided to young people who embrace those roles and spend time helping out in their community.

Assets 11–16 emphasise the importance of rules and monitoring in teenagers' lives. They emphasise *boundaries and expectations*. Research from across the world has shown that teenagers who live in families where there are clear rules exhibit lower rates of risk behaviours. It is important that adherence to these rules and expectations is monitored by parents and that consequences are in place where adolescents fall short of the expected behaviours. Similarly, young people who attend schools where there are rules and consequences are at an advantage. This asset-based approach highlights the importance of adults as role models. Teenagers learn most from what they *see* the important adults in their lives doing, particularly their parents. They will develop coping skills and strategies similar to those they see around them.

Asset 15 relates to positive peer influence. As emphasised previously, peers are a powerful influence on teenagers. While peer pressure is usually conceptualised as a negative influence, this asset reminds us it can be a healthy influence. If a teenager surrounds themself with competent, prosocial teenagers, they can have a significant protective influence on that teenager. In contrast, if an adolescent has peers who use substances, then this increases the likelihood that they will also use substances. The influence of boyfriends and girlfriends can have a similar and powerful impact.

It is also helpful if the important adults in teenagers' lives, such as parents and teachers, have high expectations of them. Obviously, if the expectations are excessively high and unattainable, this can be unhelpful. However, it seems beneficial for these adults to have expectations that are *high but manageable*. If these important adults have relatively low expectations, some teenagers will underachieve in life, especially those who lack the internal assets regarding their own intrinsic commitment to learning.

It is important for young people to make *constructive use of their time* by being given opportunities to discover talents and widen their social network in a structured and partially supervised manner. Hence, young people who are actively involved in creative activities, sport or youth organisations for a few hours every week exhibit better mental health and lower rates of risk behaviour.

Asset 19 may seem somewhat controversial in an increasingly secular Western society. It states that adolescents who are involved in religion are at an advantage. Young people who report some degree of spirituality or religiosity demonstrate lower rates of substance use, along with lower rates of aggression and deliberate self-harm. The exact mechanism of action of this particular asset is not entirely clear. However, most religions emphasise personal characteristics such as restraint and encourage young people to exhibit a caring attitude towards others, while simultaneously asking them to believe their life has a purpose. Consequently, religious affiliation may reinforce or support many of the internal assets.

The last of the external assets emphasises the importance of *spending time at home*. It has been observed in numerous studies that teenagers who spend large amounts of time with their peers 'just hanging out', exhibit significantly higher rates of risk behaviours. While it is vital that teenagers have *some* time with teenagers in such situations in order to develop basic social skills outside adult supervised settings, it is important that this does not become an everyday activity. Indeed, it is recommended that teenagers hang out with friends 'with nothing special to do' for no more than 2 evenings per week.

SPECIFIC PROTECTIVE FACTORS AGAINST ALCOHOL INITIATION AND ABUSE

Parents and teenage drinking

As a general rule, parents underestimate their influence on their children. This may be a reaction to the reduction in their influence, which does occur at the onset of adolescence. As people enter their teenage years, they become more open to influence by peers, media and popular culture. When they begin to discover their own sense of values and ideas, they will often discard some of their parents' beliefs for a period of time. Some teenagers will tell parents bluntly that they don't care what they think, most often in the context of an argument. It is important that parents do not catastrophise this reduction in influence. Indeed, *it seems fairly clear that parents remain the biggest single influence on their adolescents' behaviour and decision-making throughout the teenage years.*

A negative consequence of parents' underestimating their influence is that they can opt out of parenting if they believe their efforts are ineffective. It is important that parents don't do this. If they cease *trying* to exert a positive influence, the other elements of influence become increasingly powerful and those elements may not be as supportive, depending upon the type of environment the teenager finds themself in.

Australian researchers conducted a review of the international research on parental factors influencing teenage drinking.[6] They explored parenting factors associated with delaying the initiation of drinking and reducing alcohol-related harm in adolescents. Six factors were associated with both outcomes. Two factors were related directly to alcohol and the remaining four related to general parenting. The factors were:

- parental drinking increases risk
- provision of alcohol by parents to their children increased risk
- presence of clear rules in the family home reduced risk
- parental monitoring of their children's activities reduced risk
- warmth in the relationship between parents and children reduced risk
- general positive communication between parents and children reduced risk.

Therefore, it is a bad idea for parents to give alcohol to their children. Unfortunately, many well-intentioned and highly educated parents do this in the misguided belief that it will confer some degree of protection upon their children.

Some parents engage in this behaviour because they believe that drink is commonly provided to teenagers in many Mediterranean cultures, yet the adults in these cultures exhibit relatively low rates of risky drinking. Unfortunately, this logic is somewhat perverse and is attributing causality in the wrong direction. In Anglo-Saxon cultures, where adults' drinking episodes frequently end up as drunken episodes, the provision of alcohol to teenagers appears to hurtle them into this binge drinking culture at an earlier age. People in Mediterranean cultures *can* let adolescents drink alcohol *because* adults drink in such a low-risk manner and because *drunkenness is almost universally condemned* in those cultures. While often misrepresented as being liberal, the Mediterranean approach to alcohol is actually extremely conservative in its view of intoxication.

In Anglo-Saxon culture, adolescents who are given alcohol in supervised settings exhibit higher rates of alcohol-related harm and problems than those young people who are not given drink in a supervised manner. This fact was demonstrated in an elegant study by Barbara McMorris and colleagues[7] conducted in Australia and the United States, two cultures with quite differing views on adolescent drinking. It appears that teenagers who are given permission to drink by their parents will often drink in a restrained manner while in their parents' company. However, the same teenagers also then give *themselves* permission to drink in other social situations with their peers. They are less restrained in those circumstances than teenagers who know they are not permitted to drink under any conditions.

Another problem with parents permitting a teenager to drink relates to those teenagers who run into obvious subsequent difficulties. Having allowed the teenager to drink under supervision, it is hard to reign in that freedom once it emerges that the teenager is abusing alcohol in a problematic manner.

The review by Ryan and colleagues[6] confirmed the importance of family boundaries. Young people who report having clear rules in their family with definite consequences when they are breached have been shown to demonstrate lower rates of alcohol misuse.[2] In general terms, it appears to be beneficial for parents to have a small number of household rules that are consistently enforced, rather than lots of rules which are harder to monitor. The magnitude of the sanction for breaching rules does not need to be severe. It is simply important that it is implemented consistently when rules are broken.

The fourth factor, and perhaps linked to the last factor, relates to parental monitoring of their adolescent's activities. Teenagers who say that their parents have a good idea about where they are, who they are with and what they are doing, demonstrate significantly reduced risk of alcohol problems during adolescence.

The final two factors relate to the first two developmental assets. Generally, it is observed that young people who describe a warm and affectionate relationship with parents are less inclined to abuse alcohol. Finally, young people who report positive communication with their parents are at reduced risk. Interestingly, in terms of relative importance, the boundaries and expectations (i.e. elements of demandingness as outlined in Figure 2.1) appear to have a more powerful influence than the loving relationship and close communication (i.e. responsiveness).[2,8] Unfortunately, many parents prioritise the latter and choose not to have clear rules for fear of damaging their 'friendship' with their child, opting for the unhelpful laissez-faire style of parenting described in Chapter 2.[9] Good communication and a loving relationship with parents are shown to be ineffective in reducing alcohol misuse in the absence of simultaneous presence of rules and monitoring. Therefore, parents should prioritise these tougher elements of parenting.

Of lesser, but still significant, importance is the warm relationship and good communication between mentor and apprentice. If parents have a warm and affectionate relationship with good communication, it is easier to put rules in place and to monitor adherence to these.

'Controlled' adolescent drinking?

There are a significant minority of parents who attempt to manage this problem by permitting it. Similarly, there are some professionals who argue that this approach should be adopted. From a professional perspective, this seems to be an extension and probable misinterpretation of the 'harm reduction' approach, which has been successful in other areas of substance abuse treatment. While harm reduction is a useful and evidence-based model in the *treatment* of individuals who have a significant substance use problem, it is simply not effective as a core pillar of a *prevention* strategy. Rather than being a true harm reduction approach, giving alcohol to teenagers could be more accurately decribed as an attempt at 'managed harm escalation'.

We are unaware of any benefits of drinking in this age range. The evidence to date indicates that efforts to manage the problem by permitting it have failed.[6,7] In work with adolescents and their parents, we suggest that you also support this view that *drinking should be delayed in adolescence for as long as possible.* In practice, this probably means encouraging parents to adhere to the age at which drink can legally be purchased by their child and to discourage parents from permitting or providing drinking opportunities for their teenagers prior to this.

While the advice by the surgeon general in the United States has been unequivocal in this regard,[10] we perceive the advice of the chief medical officer in England to be unhelpful.[11] This latter document stated clearly that children under 15 years old should not drink. However, it stated that while abstinence was 'the healthiest option' for 15- to 17-year-olds, they could drink albeit with a multitude of caveats regarding quantity, frequency and supervision. This complex and muddled message has only added to confusion among parents and professionals alike. It ignores the evidence. Many people have concluded from this advice that it is okay for 15-year-olds to drink.

Now we will outline the counterarguments to the points made by people who propose permitting or accepting underage drinking.

- *'They are going to drink anyway, so it is pointless to prohibit it.'*
  This statement is partly true. In Anglo-Saxon cultures most young people drink alcohol before they have reached an age that they can legally purchase it. However, it is wrong to conclude from this fact that we should permit drinking. In reality, teenagers do *many* things we wish they would not do.

  Indeed, young children also do many things that we wish they would not do. Parents will be familiar with the reality that children aged 6–8 years often get into fights with one another. Indeed, most parents would acknowledge that almost every child of that age will occasionally get into a fight and will physically hit out at siblings. Nevertheless, we would view it as preposterous for those parents to conclude from this fact that they will therefore permit kicking and punching because the behaviour was inevitable.

Most young adolescents will occasionally choose not to do a particular element of their homework. Again, most rational people would view it as preposterous to conclude that parents and teachers therefore should allow children to opt out of homework. The fact that breaching a rule is highly likely does not mean there is no place for the rule. Indeed, the opposite is probably true. It is pointless to have rules for behaviours that never occur. It is the common behaviours that *require* rules.

- *'I don't want them drinking in fields with friends. I would rather they had a couple of drinks under my supervision.'*
  This view ignores the reality that most people choose to drink with their peers, whether they are adolescents or adults. Just because a teenager may agree to have a couple of beers with their parents does not mean that they will refuse to drink in a park or someone else's house when their parents are not around to provide supervision. Indeed, research indicates that they are more likely to drink in these unsupervised settings if you have already given them permission to drink at home.[7]

- *'Teenagers just want to rebel, if you tell them not to drink it will make them want to drink even more.'*
  Most teenagers are reasonable and sensible. It is only a minority who are intrinsically rebellious. If this statement were really correct, then it would be pointless to have any rules. Parents who permit drinking for this reason will presumably have a rule that they don't want their teenagers to stab people, snort cocaine or steal. If parents genuinely believe that teenagers will automatically choose to do things that adults tell them not to do, then they should obviously permit all of these antisocial activities.

- *'By me giving them just two bottles of beer, it puts me in charge of their drinking. It's better than me doing nothing.'*
  Most parents are aware of the dangers of hazardous drinking and want to take steps to address this problem. We are attracted to an idea that we can control it by seeking to manage it. Unfortunately, the evidence does not support this view.[6,7] At the end of the day, parents who permit drinking end up having more rules than parents who do not permit drinking in any circumstance. The tolerant parents ends up with a rule about the type of alcohol (e.g. banning spirits), another rule about the volume of alcohol that can be consumed (e.g. no more than three bottles of beer), another rule about the places where alcohol is consumed and rules about who must be present when drinking occurs (e.g. only in the presence of parents). A teenager may have three bottles of beer at home under supervision and then go out with friends to a party. If they return 3 hours later appearing a little intoxicated, what can the parent really conclude? The teenager can argue they had nothing further to drink and that it is the after effects of alcohol

that they consumed at home. The parent cannot know for sure that this is not the case. Therefore, the home-based drinking provides camouflage for additional 'top up' drinking.

RISK AND PROTECTIVE FACTORS FOR DRUG ABUSE
Family and community factors

Additional factors that increase the likelihood that a teenager commences drug use include the use of drugs by older siblings or parents. This again highlights the importance of parental modelling. While acceptance of drug use is not nearly as prevalent as acceptance of teenage drinking, it does occasionally occur. It may have its origin in the fact that parents smoked cannabis as teenagers or that they have come to believe that their teenager's assertion that 'everyone is smoking cannabis nowadays' is true. In either case, this parental tolerance is unhelpful and parents are better off holding a position that they will not permit drug use by their adolescent.

Many studies have indicated that teenagers who grow up in single parent families are more likely to develop substance use problems. This is probably a reflection of the challenges involved in parenting in general. It is easier where the parenting tasks can be shared between two people, rather than falling entirely on the shoulders of one parent. However, while parenting alone brings more challenges it can certainly be done successfully.

Dangers of early school leaving

School provides an environment in which teenagers can develop and practise their growing repertoire of positive social skills. Children who find themselves out of school are at a very significant disadvantage. There is a wealth of research that indicates that early school leaving is associated with a range of negative outcomes. Such teenagers are more likely to head towards delinquency and to become involved in crime, possibly ending up incarcerated. They are more likely to be unemployed, to become a teenage parent and to be confined to poorly paid jobs. They are also more likely to develop serious substance use problems.

In recent decades, most Western countries have put in place a broader range of educational settings for adolescents who struggle with the standard senior school environment. This is certainly a positive development as these educational settings provide an environment where the young person can access ongoing learning, but, equally important, provide an environment where there is a greater likelihood that they will develop the useful prosocial skills that are typically obtained in the ordinary school setting.

Unfortunately by the time a teenager becomes dependent upon drugs like heroin or cocaine, they are generally out of the educational system, usually with no qualifications. If they are in a Western country, they are likely to find themselves in a place where the job market for unskilled uneducated youngsters has completely contracted compared with 30 years ago. They are thus at a huge disadvantage to their peers, even if or when they overcome their drug problem.

In terms of community influences, if there is widespread availability and use of drugs within a community then teenagers are certainly at increased risk of experimenting and of developing more problematic patterns of use. Severe drug problems appear more common in deprived communities. Drugs go in and out of fashion and society often finds itself reacting to new challenges after a problem has become quite entrenched.

Extensive use of drugs such as cocaine, amphetamine and heroin can become normalised in certain communities for periods of time. Deprived communities which experience high rates of unemployment, poorer educational attainment and more criminal activity are most vulnerable to descending into these phases. Young people in those communities have fewer external assets as a result of that deprivation. A teenager in that community may quite easily drift into a serious drug problem, especially if they have less than average internal assets, despite the efforts of their family. See a brief summary of this phenomenon in Dublin in the 1990s in Box 5.1.

BOX 5.1 Heroin and Dublin in the 1990s

Most people grow up in communities largely devoid of heroin. We may find it hard to believe that someone could possibly just drift into something as dreadfully serious as heroin use. We need to understand the context in which some teenagers grow up. A heroin 'epidemic' swept across Dublin in the 1990s.[12] Dublin had the youngest population of heroin users in Europe at the end of that decade. There were six or seven hotspots for heroin use, all of which were communities with longstanding and severe deprivation. If you were male and 15 years old living in one of those communities in 1993, you had a one in five chance of becoming heroin addicted by the time you were 20. Heroin use became almost part of the normal adolescent experience of growing up. Fortunately, a decade later, due in part to the success of a National Drugs Strategy, the incidence of heroin addiction in those communities is now a small fraction of those levels.

Specific individual risk factors for substance use disorders
Embracing the drug user identity
We have noted a challenging phenomenon with regard to cannabis users in particular. A significant segment of cannabis users view cannabis as central to

their identity, with almost religious fervour. They embrace a cannabis using lifestyle, arguing that it is harmless or actually helpful, placing great weight on the fact that it is 'natural'. They contend that more people should smoke it and that society should legalise it. They are often well informed about the politics around cannabis. Such teenagers are frequently intelligent and articulate. While this is probably not unique to cannabis, it does seem to be a more common feature of that particular cohort. Users of amphetamines, cocaine or heroin will rarely define themselves in a positive way by their use of this substance. However, people who were part of the rave culture back in the 1990s tend to be happy to define themselves as such and viewed their use of stimulant drugs like ecstasy as central to their identity at that time.

Where a person is embracing drug use as a core part of their identity and viewing this positively, it poses an additional challenge when working with them to reduce or cease that use, even if they acknowledge it is causing problems in their lives. Therefore, where a teenager begins to align themselves to a subculture or a counterculture among whom drug use is seen as a defining characteristic, this poses a significant risk factor for developing problematic use of that substance and makes that individual more resistant to treatment.

Money

Teenagers who have the most money, typically sourced from parents, are more likely to drift into problematic substance use. Drink and drugs are relatively expensive commodities. Those with cash can afford to buy more regularly and in larger quantities. Consequently, experimentation can more easily progress to problematic use.

Mental health problems

Teenagers with certain mental health problems are more likely to develop substance use problems. Not all mental health problems increase risk. The specific mental health problems that are of most concern are conduct disorder, attention deficit hyperactivity disorder (ADHD) and psychotic disorders.

Conduct disorder affects about 5% of adolescents and is more common in boys.[13] It is marked by a tendency to engage in antisocial behaviours including violence, stealing, lying and cheating. These behaviours cause problems at home, at school and with peers. Some children show these behaviours from early childhood, while in others, they only emerge in adolescence. While both groups show very elevated levels of substance use, it is the group who are conduct disordered from childhood who are most at risk. Children with ADHD are at increased risk of abusing substances during adolescence. Effective treatment of the ADHD with medication appears to reduce this risk back to normal levels. ADHD greatly increases the risk that a person will have conduct disorder.

It is this relationship with conduct disorder that explains the elevated risk of substance abuse.[14] Teenagers with ADHD without a coexisting conduct disorder are probably *not* at increased risk of substance use problems, apart from cigarette smoking.

There has been long-standing debate about the relationship between substance use and psychotic disorders. It has been noted that teenagers with schizophrenia show elevated levels of substance use, especially cannabis. As discussed in Chapter 4, it is now generally accepted that adolescent cannabis use increases risk of subsequent development of schizophrenia. It also appears that teenagers with illnesses like schizophrenia are more likely to abuse drugs like cannabis. They do so for a range of reasons including relief of boredom and short-term relief of anxiety or symptoms such as hearing voices. Whatever the motivations for use, teenagers with schizophrenia who use drugs are difficult to treat and have poor outcomes, both in terms of their mental illness and their substance use. They require coordinated care shared across mental health services and substance abuse services.

Genetics

It is clear that genetic factors contribute to the risk for development of serious substance use disorders. Most of the genetic studies to date have focused on alcohol. The genetic component of alcohol dependence was initially established via adoption and twin studies. These studies confirmed that adopted children with an alcohol dependent biological parent, had increased risk of dependence themselves when they reached adulthood. The twin studies reveal higher rates of concordance between identical twins compared to non-identical twins. If a biological parent has a history of dependence, then their offspring have a two to three-fold increase in risk of dependence. Importantly, despite the increase in risk, most of their children will not grow up to develop dependence. While efforts have been made to identify specific genes that increase the risk of dependence, studies have not demonstrated consistent outcomes. There is evidence for a genetic component to some characteristics such as impulse control. Also, people may differ in their brain's reactivity to the dopamine-enhancing effect of substances.[15] This variation in dopamine activity is likely to have a genetic basis.

CASE VIGNETTE

Here we have outlined a case vignette that describes a young person who has developed significant substance use problems. We encourage you to read this vignette, noting which Assets are present and which are absent.

Case example

Nick is 18 and has been attending a specialist treatment service for heroin-addicted teenagers. Nick is easy to like, he's pleasant, calm and chatty. Prior to treatment he was smoking heroin for 15 months. He injected a few times but this frightened him. He always swore he would never inject, looking down on injectors as 'scumbags'. He began drinking at age 12 and commenced smoking cannabis soon after. He preferred the 'mellow buzz' of cannabis and disliked the hangovers and blackouts that came with alcohol. He used ecstasy intermittently from age 14 and occasionally used cocaine at this time. He began smoking heroin the odd weekend at 15. The first few times he used heroin, it was to come down off ecstasy and cocaine, after a night out partying. He loved the way heroin made him feel.

Although Nick has always had some income through jobs over the last couple of years, he had to supplement this money in the months prior to starting treatment. He robbed cars and shoplifted. He's never been charged and had avoided getting into debt. Nick lives with his parents and has three older brothers. His 25-year-old brother also used heroin and attends the local clinic for treatment. Nick's two oldest brothers left school early. Nick and his mother could name 10 young adults on their street who had heroin problems.

Nick's mother reports that he was 'an average baby'. At playschool he was perceived to be a good mixer. In junior school, Nick did not experience problems, despite rarely doing his homework. There were never too many rules at home and his mum found him easy to manage. She worried when he started staying out overnight with friends but she thought his friends were generally 'nice lads'. After these overnight events, his mother tried to explain to him the dangers associated with his lifestyle, but he didn't seem to care.

He disliked senior school from the outset. Most of his friends from junior school had gone to different schools. He didn't like the new subjects. Despite this, he did not get into any substantial difficulty. He got on reasonably well with teachers. He was offered some work with his uncle during his third year of senior school and he decided to leave education. He thought he could always go back to school the next year if things didn't work out. After six months, his uncle's business became quieter and he was let go. He started in an alternative education setting for early school leavers but this was in a different neighbourhood. He felt like he had nothing in common with the other lads there and thought they were a bit 'stuck up'. For these reasons, he dropped out. Since then, Nick had a number of different jobs. Oftentimes the work was casual and short-term. However, there were a few jobs he just left. When Nick decided to discontinue a particular job, his mother was generally supportive and understanding of these decisions.

Like most heroin-addicted teenagers we have met, Nick simply drifted out of school. Very few have been expelled due to major discipline difficulties. It seems that these children, particularly those from deprived communities, were surrounded by a poverty of expectation. By this we mean that it was often the case that neither teenager, parent, nor school held any real expectation that they would remain in education (absence of assets 5, 16, 21 and 24).

These adolescents rarely had any great expectation for their own future (assets 37 and 40). Their parents' ambivalence towards education may be due to the fact that many of them found the inflexible educational system they experienced to be difficult. Equally they may have found that educational success didn't necessarily lead to increased employment opportunities during times of recession and financial difficulty. Despite legislation requiring children to remain in education until their mid-teenage years, all too often, some schools seem willing to let these teenagers drift away.

As in Nick's case, this early departure from school is often followed by affiliation with an older and substance-abusing peer group. They gradually progressed from alcohol to cannabis to taking tablets and on to smoking heroin. Almost before they knew it, they were 'strung out'.

CONCLUSION

In their eloquent and comprehensive review of this topic Cicchetti and Rogosch[16] emphasise that there are a great many potential routes into addiction. The journey to that point typically involves the interplay of psychological, family, school, community and cultural factors. An understanding of the common risk and protective factors allows for the development and implementation of prevention strategies and can guide treatment interventions.

KEY POINTS

- While there are many routes into substance use among adolescents, many risk and protective factors have been identified. These occur in the biological, psychological, family, school, community and cultural domains.
- Recently, there has been a shift in focus from risk factors to protective assets.
- Many of the factors that reduce the risk of developing a substance problem also reduce risk of other mental health and behavioural issues, and vice versa.
- Parents are a powerful influence on adolescents, yet they frequently underestimate their influence. An authoritative parenting style is most protective.

- Parental provision of alcohol to adolescents increases risk of harmful drinking.
- Early school leaving, peer substance use and community deprivation each contributes to risk.

FURTHER READING

➡ *40 Developmental Assets*: the Search Institute's website (www.search-institute.org) is the online home of the 40 Developmental Assets. The site is particularly suited to professionals.

➡ Ungar M, Ghazinour M, Richter J. What is resilience within the social ecology of human development? *J Child Psychol Psychiatry.* 2013; **54**(4): 348–66.

REFERENCES

1 Leffert N, Benson PL, Scales PC, *et al.* Developmental assets: measurement and prediction of risk behaviors among adolescents. *Appl Dev Sci.* 1998; **2**(4): 209–30.

2 McKay MT, Sumnall H, Goudie AJ, *et al.* What differentiates adolescent problematic drinkers from their peers? Results from a cross-sectional study in Northern Irish school children. *Drug-Educ Prev Polic.* 2011; **18**(3): 187–99.

3 Mischel W, Ayduk O, Berman MG, *et al.* 'Willpower' over the life span: decomposing self-regulation. *Soc Cogn Affect Neurosci.* 2011; **6**(2): 252–6.

4 Rotter JB. External control and internal control. *Psychol Today.* 1971; **5**(1): 37–42.

5 Ashton M. Confident kids . . . like to party. *Drugs Alcohol Findings.* 2004; 11(Autumn): 22–3. Available at: http://findings.org.uk/docs/Ashton_M_30.pdf

6 Ryan SM, Jorm AF, Lubman DI. Parenting factors associated with reduced alcohol use: a systematic review of longitudinal research. *Aust N Z J Psychiatry.* 2010; **44**(9): 774–83.

7 McMorris BJ, Catalano RF, Kim MJ, *et al.* Influence of family factors and supervised alcohol use on adolescent alcohol use and harms: similarities between youth in different alcohol policy contexts. *J Stud Alcohol Drugs.* 2011; **72**(3): 418–28.

8 Hayes L, Smart D, Toumbourou JW, *et al. Parental Influences on Adolescent Alcohol Use.* Melbourne: Australian Institute of Family Studies; 2004.

9 Department of Children, Schools and Families (DCSF). *Use of Alcohol Among Children and Young People.* London: DCSF; 2008.

10 Office of the Surgeon General. *The Surgeon General's Call to Action to Prevent and Reduce Underage Drinking.* Rockville, MD: US Department of Health and Human Services / Office of the Surgeon General; 2007.

11 Chief Medical Officer for England. *Guidance on the Consumption of Alcohol by Children and Young People.* London: Department of Health; 2009.

12 Smyth B, O'Brien M. Children attending addiction treatment services in Dublin, 1990–1999. *Eur Addict Res.* 2004: **10**(2): 68–74.

13 Maughan B, Rowe R, Messer J, *et al.* Conduct disorder and oppositional defiant

disorder in a national sample: developmental epidemiology. *J Child Psychol Psychiatry.* 2004; **45**(3): 609–21.

14 Molina BSG, Pelham WE. Childhood predictors of adolescent substance use in a longitudinal study of children with ADHD. *J Abnorm Psychol.* 2003; **112**(3): 497–507.

15 Le Foll B, Gallo A, Le Strat Y, *et al.* Genetics of dopamine receptors and drug addiction: a comprehensive review. *Behav Pharmacol.* 2009; **20**(1): 1–17.

16 Cicchetti D, Rogosch FA. Psychopathology as risk for adolescent substance use disorders: a developmental psychopathology perspective. *J Clin Child Psychol.* 1999; **28**(3): 355–65.

CHAPTER 6

Preventing adolescent substance use

INTRODUCTION

Much is written about preventing health problems. This is based on the old adage that prevention is better than cure. In healthcare, this is true and applies equally as well to substance use. Naturally those who never use substances do not suffer the harms associated with it. While it is ideal to get teenagers to never use substances, the reality is that this will never be perfectly achieved. As discussed previously, surveys around the world suggest that a significant number of children in their mid-teens have already tried drugs, with cannabis, alcohol and tobacco the most frequently used. The 2009–10 Health Behaviour of School Children Report found that 17% of students had tried cannabis, with boys more likely to do so than girls (*see* Box 6.1).[1] And while Canada topped the chart, the United States, France, Spain and the UK all reported rates of cannabis use that were above average. It's important to bear in mind that those who use drugs at a younger age are more likely to suffer related harm and have more severe problems than those who do not start their substance use until their late teens. For this reason, prevention should be seen to have two goals:

1 preventing adolescents from ever using substances in the first place
2 delaying the age of onset of drug use.

Figure 6.1 presents the impact of two hypothetical prevention approaches to cannabis initiation. Prior to any prevention intervention, it can be seen that experimentation with cannabis rises rapidly in mid-adolescence, with 26% using by age 15 years and 42% by age 20 years. With prevention strategy A, this results in a delay in onset of experimentation (only 16% have tried cannabis by age 15 years), but the overall proportion who use by age 20 years is unchanged. Given the hazards associated with early-onset cannabis use, this is still a positive impact. However, prevention strategy B has a more profound impact, causing a delay in onset of use and also resulting in less experimentation overall by the age of 20 years.

BOX 6.1 Research review

The Health Behaviour of School-aged Children (HBSC) study is an international project that researches the various health-related behaviours across children in numerous countries. Behaviours examined include diet, exercise and leisure activity, as well as tobacco and substance use. It is completed every 4 years and allows for comparisons not just between countries but also across time. For example, the HSBC mean for rates of 15-year-olds who smoke tobacco at least once a week was 19% in 2005–06 but 18% in 2009–10. A small change in the right direction. When we examine the HBSC data for England, we see that in 2005 18% of girls and 13% of boys smoked weekly at the age of 15. By 2009, the figures had reduced to 14% and 9%, respectively. This indicates that positive changes are being made in England regarding smoking.

Another important issue is the fact that each substance an adolescent uses makes them more likely to use another. This has important implications for the prevention of substance use. Someone who smokes cigarettes is more likely to use cannabis than someone who doesn't. Likewise, someone who drinks is more likely to try another intoxicating substance. Smoking tobacco and drinking alcohol are the most common substances used by teenagers throughout the world. For this reason, society needs to take them seriously, not just because of

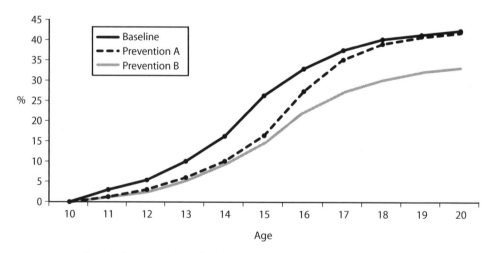

FIGURE 6.1 Cumulative proportion of adolescents who have experimented with cannabis

the harm they cause themselves but also because anything that reduces alcohol and tobacco use is also likely to reduce the use of other drugs.[2]

There is an important aspect of research that comes into play when trying to prevent any particular problem: the concept of causality. It is relatively easy in research to identify whether there is a relationship between two variables. For example, research has repeatedly shown that people who begin drinking early in adolescence are more likely to use cocaine as adults.[2] The *gateway theory* suggests that these events are causally related. Another theory is the *common liability model*.[3] It suggests that use of one drug does not directly cause use of other substances. However, people who lack a number of protective factors or assets (*see* Table 5.1) are more likely to drink early and more likely to use cocaine as young adults. The gateway theory and the common liability model are often presented as *competing* explanations. Of course, they *may both be true*, given the heterogeneity of routes to cocaine use as an adult. People who drink in early adolescence and use cocaine as young adults are not all the same. For many, both behaviours will have their origins in the lack of assets (i.e. consistent with the common liability model). For others, the early drinking may have caused a psychological, neurobiological or social change, which in turn made them more likely to use cocaine later.

Things that have an impact on substance use by teens can be divided into two categories: risk and protective factors (*see* Chapter 5). In working at preventing substance use problems, the goal is to maximise protective and minimise risk factors. Unfortunately it is not possible to guarantee a particular child will not use drugs or alcohol. There is no single thing (or combination of things for that matter) that guarantees someone will never have a problem. Much like cancer prevention, we can only play the odds – all parents, or others working with teenagers, can do is put in place as many protective factors and remove as many risk factors as possible (*see* Figure 5.1). Frequently, we meet parents and professionals who refuse to accept the research evidence and rely on their own opinions. While writing this book we have reviewed much of the literature on this area and are thus presenting the best research evidence.

In this chapter we will explore strategies to put in place protective factors. For convenience we will divide them into related areas such as school, parents and peers. One thing to bear in mind is that risk factors tend to be the same across a variety of health-related behaviours. Teenagers who use drugs are also more likely to drink alcohol, smoke tobacco, skip school and have sex earlier. Therefore, many interventions that protect a teenager from drug use are also likely to have a positive impact on school dropout and vice versa.

UNDERSTANDING HEALTH PROMOTION

Health promotion is the branch of healthcare related to promoting good health and avoiding disease. It is hard to discuss preventing adolescent substance use without at least mentioning health promotion. Traditionally health promotion is broken into three categories.

1 *Primary health promotion* is concerned with the prevention of problems before they start. The effort to stop people from commencing smoking cigarettes is a good example of this. Banning illicit drugs is another example.

2 *Secondary health promotion* accepts that, in some cases, people will have developed health problems and so the focus is on eradicating them, ideally before major harm comes. This includes efforts to get people to stop smoking. For substance use, it could include counselling for those who are using.

3 *Tertiary health promotion* is synonymous with harm minimisation in substance abuse treatment. Tertiary strategies are reserved for when it is not possible to prevent the problem. Smoking bans that reduce opportunities for people to smoke fall into this category, as does the provision of needle exchange facilities to drug users. The aim is to minimise the harm done by the disease or behaviour.

In this chapter, much of what we discuss falls into the primary category and, to a lesser extent, the secondary category. Substance abuse treatment strategies such as counselling, medications and family therapy fall within the secondary and tertiary areas, as they are generally focused on working with someone who is already using substances. However, a 16-year-old receiving counselling to reduce the harm associated with his cannabis use (a tertiary-level intervention) could also receive interventions to ensure he does not progress to using heroin. This heroin-related intervention could be seen as a primary prevention strategy.

Figure 6.2 outlines the levels of intervention diagrammatically. Without intervention there is a tendency for people to move clockwise across categories of use. Some people will also spontaneously move anticlockwise, or become abstinent. Various health promotion interventions seek to actively intervene in this process, by blocking movement in a clockwise direction (i.e. escalations in use) and by causing movement in an anticlockwise direction (i.e. reductions in use).

Programmes aimed at preventing substance use can be targeted in three ways. The first are *universal interventions*, which are delivered to all. Typically this includes school-based interventions where every child in the school receives the intervention. Most Western countries provide a variety of universal health programmes to schoolchildren on a variety of topics including substance use. *Selective interventions* are interventions that are targeted at risk

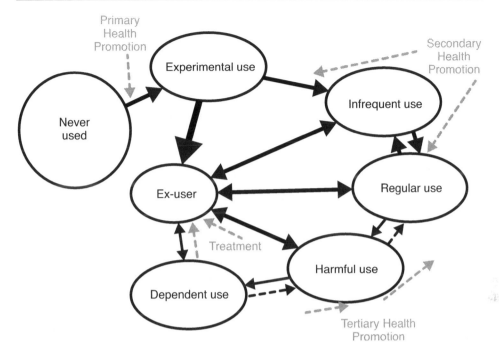

FIGURE 6.2 Health promotion and adolescent substance use

groups or subgroups of the general population. For example, children in disadvantaged areas may get additional interventions targeting particular risks. Finally, *indicated interventions* are targeted at subgroups who have already demonstrated substance use problems or are showing evidence of progression to substance use.

FAMILY-FOCUSED SUBSTANCE USE PREVENTION

Evidence indicates that parents are the most important influence on teenagers (*see* Chapter 5). Many parents feel powerless as their children grow up and consequently they sometimes underestimate the influence they have. In other cases, parents are overly confident about what their children are doing and therefore don't realise they are using substances. Almost every evidence-based treatment for adolescent substance use involves some work with parents.

Despite this growing scientific understanding of the power of parental influence and identification of the specific parenting strategies that are helpful in reducing teenage drinking, there has been little success in communicating this information to parents. Research from Britain, Australia and Ireland suggests that many parents are confused about what to do and many feel disempowered in addressing teenage drinking.[4-6]

As discussed in Chapter 5, Ryan, *et al.*[7] found it was important for parents to adhere to an authoritative parenting style (i.e. have household rules, monitor their adolescent's lifestyle and to maintain positive communication and a warm relationship). They also found that both parental drinking and parental provision of alcohol to adolescents increased risk.

Unfortunately, in many Western countries, it seems many parents have become more permissive, and perceive themselves as having reduced ability to control their children.[8] There is evidence of an interaction between parenting style and intrinsic adolescent characteristics.[4,9] The impact of poor parenting practice tends to be most detrimental to adolescents who lack the internal protective factors (e.g. impulse control and academic ambition) than it is to adolescents who have these assets.

In Sweden, a brief prevention program (the Örebro Prevention Program) that encouraged parents to maintain strict attitudes towards teenage drinking successfully reduced drunkenness and delinquency.[10] The intervention was relatively simple. Staff from the programme attended parent–teacher meetings and discussed ways in which parents could encourage their teens to get involved in activities and to get the parents to write and sign written copies of their position on drinking. In addition, information on leisure activities were posted to all parents along with information on maintaining strict alcohol rules. However, when the same intervention was conducted in the Netherlands, a country with a very different cultural and policy approach to alcohol use, the programme did not reduce teenage drinking. This may indicate that such programmes do not work or it may indicate that it is unrealistic to expect a parent-based intervention to successfully transplant from one culture to another. However, a recent Cochrane Review of parent and family prevention interventions, many of which were complex and intensive, demonstrated their effectiveness in reducing adolescent alcohol problems.[11,12]

Specific advice for parents

In this section, we offer readers general tips about what parents can do to reduce the likelihood that their child will develop substance use problems.[7] We hope these ideas can be used by those working with parents to offer some guidance about what advice to give. The following items are not placed in any order of importance and should be viewed as equally important. Ideally, parents should be implementing these strategies prior to adolescence.

1 Monitor where teenagers are and who they are with

As children get older they often change friends. Parents should demonstrate an interest in their children's lifestyle. Many children who start using substances move into a group of friends who also use. Similarly, when someone has friends who commence substance use this increases their chances of doing so. Parents can make efforts to get to know their children's friends and where they spend their time. Have they changed their friends? What are their friends like? Do you know their friends' parents? It is also worth thinking about where they hang out.

2 Have healthy communication

Parents need to maintain their important role in their child's life. Being overly authoritarian and critical can lead to a situation where children feel alienated and this reduces the likelihood that they will talk to their parents about their worries. Good communication is vital. Parents should comment on and affirm children's positive behaviour. However, simply avoiding conflict is not healthy. Parents need to strike a balance between letting children know what behaviours are and are not acceptable and having fun with them.

3 Be a good role model

Research has shown that children who see their parents drinking, smoking or using drugs are more likely to follow suit. This can be challenging in many countries where alcohol is seen as a normal part of culture. When adolescents enter substance use treatment, many models suggest advising parents to remove alcohol/drugs from the home and avoid using around their children.

4 Have clear and appropriate rules

A parent's job is to parent: they are in charge and rules are necessary. Consequences need to be in place when children break rules. Some children are naturally more responsible and mature and so the rules may need to be adapted for each child in the same family. If a child wants freedom to stay out later they need to demonstrate they can handle this extra freedom responsibly. It does not make sense to give incremental freedoms to a teenager who is constantly getting in trouble simply because they are now 16!

5 Address drugs and alcohol directly

We believe parents should make it clear to their children that substance use is not permitted. They should explain to their child why they hold this position. It is because the risks substantially outweigh the benefits. The clearer the rules parents hold around this the better. Just because a child breaks a rule and drinks does not mean the rule has failed. A more tolerant and permissive attitude has repeatedly been shown to lead to more drinking or drug use.

6 Free time and hobbies

Using drugs takes up time. Teenagers with more free time are more likely to use drugs. Parents can work at keeping their children occupied. The more involved with school and leisure activities a child is, the less likely they are to develop a problem. Parents can actively facilitate their child to get involved with activities such as sport, youth projects, music, art and drama. Fundamentally, it is not important which activity is chosen – the goal is to find something the child likes to do. Bear in mind that it is not possible for children to spend all of their free time at clubs. It is normal for teens to just hang out. We suggest that a limit is set on the amount of time the teenager can spend out with friends just hanging out. Boxes 6.2 and 6.3 provide some examples of focused prevention approaches.

BOX 6.2 The Home Party Approach[13]

One of the challenges in prevention work is how get the information out to parents. A group of researchers in the Netherlands came up with a novel approach to this dilemma. Called the Home Party Approach, it is similar to the idea of a 'Tupperware party'. The prevention worker recruits a host parent who agrees to hold a 2-hour session in his or her home on preventing substance use problems in children. The host parent then recruits other parents and the prevention worker delivers a workshop to the parents in the host parent's house.

BOX 6.3 Strengthening Families Programme

The Strengthening Families Programme (SFP) is a comprehensive and intensive intervention delivered to families, typically involving fourteen 2-hour sessions. In each session, groups of parents and adolescents meet separately initially for an hour, before then joining together for larger family group sessions. The evening begins with everyone sharing a meal together. The parent sessions focus on rules, communication, rewarding healthy behaviour and accessing supports in the wider community. The adolescent sessions focus on issues such as building positive expectancies, stress management and peer relationships. As such, SFP goals are consistent with the 40 Developmental Assets Approach (*see* Chapter 5). There is evidence to indicate both short- and long-term benefits from the SFP have been demonstrated to be cost-effective. Although initially developed in the United States, the SFP has been implemented in a range of cultural settings (see www.strengtheningfamiliesprogram.org/).

PEERS AND PREVENTION

Having friends is a normal part of growing up. Whenever we discuss adolescent substance use, we hear complaints about peer pressure and the negative effect of friends. It is important to note that the effect of peers is not always negative. If students believe their friends hold negative attitudes towards intoxication or substance use, they are less likely to use. Therefore, encouraging teenagers to develop relationships and friendships with peers who do not use drugs and who disapprove of it would be helpful.

It is not possible for parents to pick their teenagers' friends. Trying to make someone stop seeing his or her friends or making negative comments about the friends is unlikely to be helpful. When it comes to peers, there are a number of things that are likely to be helpful.

- Provide teenagers with opportunities to mix with peers who are likely to be prosocial influences. Activities where they are mixing with different people will help with this.
- Reduce the time they have to simply hang out with teenagers who are likely to be a poor influence. Accept that you cannot ensure they never come into contact with peers who will be a bad influence.
- So often programmes are put together for 'at risk' teens. These include clubs aimed at those deemed at risk. The downside of this well-intended intervention is that troubled teens spend more time with other troubled teenagers. Unsurprisingly, this carries significant risks, with some research suggesting group preventive strategies for at-risk teens *may actually escalate substance use* and conduct problems.[14]

ROLE OF SCHOOL AND EDUCATION IN SUBSTANCE USE PREVENTION

School is a major feature of a young person's life. In most countries, education runs until the child is about 17 years old. Young people spend a significant part of their waking hours in school and so it exerts considerable influence on them. An important thing to realise is the generally positive effect school has on young people (*see* Chapter 5). Schools typically provide activities such as sport, music and drama, which are important external assets. Additionally, schools reinforce many important values (internal assets). Those who leave school early miss out on these protective assets and tend to experience poorer outcomes in a number of aspects. They are more likely to engage in a variety of antisocial behaviours such as crime and drug use. Therefore, it is important that teenagers remain in education for as long as possible. Nevertheless, drug use can happen in school and educational programmes and so a substance use policy is needed. The development of such policies is discussed in more depth in Chapter 12.

Given the protective factors associated with school, parents and society have a duty to do what they can to ensure that young people stay in school. A number of things can be done to aid this, including those outlined as follows.

Parents
- Have high expectations from early on regarding their child's engagement in education
- Encourage their children to engage with education, for example homework
- Participate as much as possible in the school community

Society
- Provide support to adolescents to stay in school
- Provide alternative education options to those who leave mainstream school early
- Have a monitoring system to ensure children get to school and deal with it when they don't
- Have a mandatory age up to which children must attend school
- Help schools deal effectively with substance use issues while keeping children in school; suspending students until they are drug free is unlikely to be effective
- Make access to substances more difficult; the most commonly used substances are naturally ones that are more available – particularly cigarettes and alcohol

Recently, efforts have been made to develop school-based drug and alcohol prevention programmes. While such programmes are popular with parents and politicians, the programme evaluations have often been disappointing.[15] Cuijpers[16] identified certain features of the most effective school-based programmes. The best results were seen where the programme:
- was based on a proven or evidence-based approach
- has a focus on norms and commitment not to use
- involves simultaneous community input, for example parental involvement
- uses peer leaders instead of or with adults.

Foxcroft and Tsertsvadze[17] conducted a Cochrane Review of school-based interventions and found evidence for effectiveness of some programmes. The LifeSkills Training programme is one example of a highly regarded programme. LifeSkills Training has been designed to be flexible and is used across most of the school-age spectrum (ages 7–17 years). The programme can be incorporated into the school curriculum over 10–30 classes. It seeks to enhance positive protective factors. It also seeks to increase awareness of drug risks and to challenge favourable attitudes to antisocial behaviour.

BOX 6.4 The Good Behaviour Game

The Good Behaviour Game is an interesting example of how simple prevention strategies can be implemented for very young children. In the first or second year of school (ages 4–6 years) students are divided into teams in the classroom for the Good Behaviour Game. Each team can then win prizes if they have fewer than four black marks against their team during a game period. Initially, game periods are short – 10- or 15-minute segments in the day – but over time the periods are extended. When followed up at around age 20, the students (particularly boys) who had been exposed to this game in their first years of school, were less likely to have substance abuse problems, to have an antisocial personality and to have been incarcerated for a violent offence.[18,19]

A recent cost-benefit analysis in the United States reports that the cost of delivering a school-based intervention to students could be as high as US$220 per student. However, they also reported that for every US$1 spent on the programme, a saving of US$18 would be made for society.[20]

In 2013, Patricia Conrod and colleagues[21] published results of an interesting school-based alcohol prevention programme. While most school-based prevention programmes are universal, their intervention was selective. They identified adolescents who demonstrated one of four predetermined risky psychological profiles, and separated them into four subgroups. They then delivered a group-based intervention over two sessions tailored to the specific psychological profile of the subgroup. The interventions were based strongly upon Motivational Interviewing and cognitive behavioural therapy (*see* Chapters 9 and 10). They demonstrated that the intervention reduced binge drinking up to 2 years after programme delivery.

HOBBIES AND INTERESTS: IMPORTANCE IN SUBSTANCE USE PREVENTION

As mentioned earlier, the more free time adolescents have, the more likely they are to have a substance abuse problem. Outside of school, the next major draw on a teenager's time is his or her hobbies. Hobbies can include:

- *sport* – including training for a sport alone or as part of an organised training session (sport does not have to be competitive and many students play informal games of basketball, soccer and baseball for fun)
- *arts* – this can include music, painting, sketching, drama and dancing
- *special interest groups* – such as Scouts, writing groups or book clubs.

When someone gets involved with a club, sport, team or music, the hobby extends much further than the time spent at the club itself. Playing music might involve a 1-hour class, but many hours are also spent practising it. The same applies to sports. Hobbies also bring a knock-on effect in relation to other protective factors. For example, forming a supportive relationship with a coach, engaging in fun and being with other teenagers who are likely to be a positive influence are additional benefits.

MENTAL HEALTH

The relationship between mental health and substance abuse is discussed in Chapter 13, but there are some key points worth making here. We know a significant relationship exists between adolescent substance use and mental health problems. Research indicates that, among teenagers attending substance abuse services, at least 50% have a mental health problem. Some studies have even suggested that this could be higher and up around 90%.[22,23]

BOX 6.5 Common mental health problems among adolescent substance users

- Mood/depressive disorders
- Deliberate self-harm
- Conduct and oppositional-defiant disorders
- Attention deficit hyperactivity disorder
- Anxiety disorders

Without question, it is vital that children with mental health problems are proactively screened for substance use. The European Monitoring Centre for Drugs and Drug Addiction has recommended that children attending mental health services be particularly targeted for substance misuse prevention work, as they are at particular risk of substance use problems.[24] For this reason, parents and mental health staff should promote activities that are likely to be helpful. It is essential that the parents of 'at-risk children' pay particular attention to the role model they provide regarding substance abuse. Given this inherent risk factor, it is important to bolster as many protective factors as possible.

THE YOUNG PERSON THEMSELF: NURTURING RESILIENCE

From a young age, children learn various ideas and attitudes from their parents, their environment and others they interact with. These ideas are not always consciously communicated but rather the child picks them up through a process of role-modelling and experience. Certain characteristics are proven to be protective from a substance use point of view. Many of these have knock-on effects in other areas such as criminality, aggression and mental health. Naturally, parents have some influence over these and should exercise this influence. As discussed earlier, school plays an important role in nurturing resilience and in providing external assets to students. Some key things to target for adolescents are outlined here.

Develop empathy and consideration

Showing empathy towards the feelings of others is important. While empathy is partly an innate characteristic, there is little doubt that the child's experience can support or hinder its development. Parents can encourage their child to be responsive to other people's feelings from a young age by getting them to think about the effect of things on others' feelings. Role-modelling is vital. If children repeatedly hear their parents being aggressive, insensitive or rude to others they will learn to do likewise.

A sense of community

Our environment is important and we all play a part in contributing to our neighbourhood – for better or worse. It is healthy for children to care for the area they live in and the people they share this with. Adults can encourage children to keep the neighbourhood tidy, help with clean-ups, getting to know neighbours and helping them as appropriate. Involvement in religious activity can also be helpful.

There are examples of large selective community-based prevention programmes internationally (e.g. SureStart in Britain).[25] These programmes have focused on deprived communities and have explicitly targeted improved outcome for children under the age of 5 years. The programmes are broad in scope but the focus is consistent with the principles outlined in the 40 Developmental Assets approach (*see* Chapter 5). It is hoped that such programmes will have a positive impact on the children who grow up in the communities where they are delivered. One of the targeted outcomes is a reduction in substance use problems for children when they reach adolescence and adulthood.

NATIONAL POLICIES TO PREVENT ALCOHOL AND DRUG PROBLEMS

Governments have a role in curtailing adolescent substance use. They can actively support families, schools and communities to adopt the strategies outlined earlier. Additionally, they can implement broad polices to reduce use of substances. Most research has been conducted on alcohol-related harm across the population and the impact of government policy on this area. The measures which reduce alcohol-related harm most effectively are those that increase the cost and restrict the availability of alcohol.[15] There is also good evidence that advertising and sponsorship encourage youth drinking.[26] Hence, many groups have advocated that alcohol promotion should be greatly curtailed or ended completely. The drinks industry powerfully and effectively opposes these measures, as they will negatively impact on profitability.[15]

Drugs policy is also increasingly a focus at the political level. Most countries ban the sale or use of almost all substances. Countries vary on the extent to which they punish or intervene with drug users. There is little evidence to guide decision-making on this issue. Many advocate a softening of legislation on drugs, such as decriminalising use. Others suggest that drug selling should be permitted. It remains to be seen how these policies will evolve and what their impact will be. Certainly many arguments in favour of legalising drugs are deeply simplistic and inaccurate. It is often stated that legalising drugs would remove criminality from the equation. However, criminal gangs have an active and lucrative trade in regulated products such as tobacco, diesel and alcohol in many countries. If other drugs are also legalised, it seems inevitable that criminal gangs will be dominant players in the drugs market. Legalising drugs is likely to result in a reduction in the cost of drugs and easier access. The lessons from alcohol indicate that these two changes will result in increased use and harm. Those who advocate making drugs legally available invariably suggest that they would not be made available to children. However, the substances that teenagers use the most are the ones that are legal but restricted from being sold to minors. If such restrictions worked, alcohol would be less, not more, frequently used than cannabis.

CONCLUSION

Our goal in this chapter was to give a sense of some things that might be useful in preventing substance use problems. While it can seem like a complicated issue, the basic idea is simple. Young people who have happy home lives, supportive families and friends, are invested in education, are caring towards others and have hobbies, are less likely to use drugs. As a bonus, they are likely to do well in a variety of other respects too. The challenge is how to provide these for a teenager. The old saying 'it takes a village to raise a child' is true. Neither one person nor one organisation can provide all that a child needs. If you have any contact with adolescents you can have an impact on the risk of them using substances (*see* Box 6.6).

BOX 6.6 Practice exercise: your role in prevention

In your role working with adolescents, is there more you could do to build resilience in the teenagers you encounter?

Are there assets that your organisation already provides?

Are there any additional assets which you or your organisation could provide?

Read again the 40 Developmental Assets and remind yourself of the important assets that foster healthy adolescent development. Tips on how to implement them are available at www.search-institute.org/content/40-developmental-assets-adolescents-ages-12-18

KEY POINTS

- The majority of teenagers do not use substances. Prevention is better than cure and so every effort should be made to prevent children from using substances.
- Guaranteeing a teenager *never* uses a substance is impossible, but there are things that can reduce the likelihood that he or she will, including school involvement, sports and hobbies, having a supportive family and clear rules.
- Accepting that some children will go on to use substances, it makes sense to focus on delaying their commencement of use. The later someone starts using a substance, the less harm they are likely to suffer.
- When a teenager is using a substance, a harm reduction focus is useful to ensure that the associated harm is limited.
- Interventions to reduce and prevent adolescent substance use can be implemented at home, school, clubs and society at large. It is everyone's responsibility.
- While families, schools, communities and individuals all have roles in preventing substance use problems, governments also play a part, particularly in the area of alcohol problems. Western governments could do more to reduce alcohol-related harm.

FURTHER READING

- *40 Developmental Assets*: the Search Institute's website (www.search-institute.org) is the home of the 40 Developmental Assets. The site is particularly suited to professionals.
- The Search Institute has developed a separate website for families and parents. Parent Further (www.parentfurther.com) provides lots of tips, articles, videos and resources that parents in particular will find useful.

⇒ *Parents Plus* (www.parentsplus.i.e.) is a programme developed in Ireland that helps parents develop the skills they need for effective parenting. It has numerous programmes including ones for parents of preschool children, children in junior school and teenagers. In addition it has a course for parents who are separated. The programme has been evaluated and has extensive evidence supporting its effectiveness.

⇒ *The Strengthening Families Program* (www.strengtheningfamiliesprogram.org) aims to develop the strengths within at-risk families. The outcomes have repeatedly demonstrated robust findings, proving it to be an effective programme.

REFERENCES

1 Currie C, Zanotti C, Morgan A, *et al.*, editors. *Social Determinants of Health and Well-Being among Young People: health behaviour in school-aged children (HBSC) study; international report from the 2009/2010 survey.* Copenhagen: World Health Organization Regional Office for Europe; 2012.

2 Fergusson DM, Boden JM, Horwood LJ. The developmental antecedents of illicit drug use: evidence from a 25-year longitudinal study. *Drug Alcohol Depend.* 2008; 96: 165–77.

3 Van Leeuwen AP, Verhulst FC, Reijneveld SA, *et al.* Can the gateway hypothesis, the common liability model and/or, the route of administration model predict initiation of cannabis use during adolescence? A survival analysis: the trails study. *J Adolesc Health.* 2011; 48(1): 73–8.

4 Hayes L, Smart D, Toumbourou JW, *et al. Parental Influences on Adolescent Alcohol Use.* Melbourne: Australian Institute of Family Studies; 2004.

5 Department of Children, Schools and Families. *Use of Alcohol among Children and Young People.* London: Department of Children, Schools and Families; 2008.

6 Van Hout MCA. Youth alcohol and drug use in rural Ireland: parents' views. *Rural Remote Health.* 2009; 9(3): 1171.

7 Ryan SM, Jorm AF, Lubman DI. Parenting factors associated with reduced alcohol use: a systematic review of longitudinal research. *Aust N Z J Psychiatry.* 2010; 44(9): 774–83.

8 Department of Health and Children. *Parents' Perspectives on Parenting Styles and Disciplining Children.* Dublin: Government Publications; 2010.

9 McKay MT, Sumnall H, Goudie AJ, *et al.* What differentiates adolescent problematic drinkers from their peers? Results from a cross-sectional study in Northern Irish school children. *Drugs-Educ Prev Polic.* 2011; 18(3): 187–99.

10 Koutakis N, Stattin H, Kerr M. Reducing youth alcohol drinking through a parent-targeted intervention: the Orebro Prevention Program. *Addiction.* 2008; 103(10): 1629–37.

11 Smit E, Verdurmen J, Monshouwer K, *et al.* Family interventions and their effect on adolescent alcohol use in general populations: a meta-analysis of randomized controlled trials. *Drug Alcohol Depend.* 2008; 97(3): 195–206.

12 Foxcroft DR, Tsertsvadze A. Universal family-based prevention programs for alcohol misuse in young people. Cochrane Database Syst Rev. 2011; 7(9): CD009308.

13 Riper H, Bolier L, Elling A. The home party: "Development of a low threshold

intervention for 'not yet reached' parents in adolescent substance use prevention". *J Subst Use.* 2005; **10**(2–3): 141–50.

14 Poulin F, Dishion TJ, Burraston B. 3-Year iatrogenic effects associated with aggregating high-risk adolescents in cognitive-behavioural preventive interventions. *Appl Dev Sci.* 2001; **5**(4): 214–24.

15 Room R, Babor T, Rehm J. Alcohol and public health. *Lancet.* 2005; **365**(9458): 519–30.

16 Cuijpers P. Effective ingredients of school-based drug prevention programs: a systematic review. *Addict Behav.* 2002; **27**(6): 1009–23.

17 Foxcroft DR, Tsertsvadze A. Universal school-based prevention programs for alcohol misuse in young people. Cochrane Database Syst Rev. 2011; **11**(5): CD009113.

18 Poduska JM, Kellam SG, Wang W, *et al.* Impact of the Good Behaviour Game, a universal classroom-based behaviour intervention, on young adult service use for problems with emotions, behaviours, or drugs or alcohol. *Drug Alcohol Depend.* 2008; **95**(Suppl. 1): S29–44.

19 Kellam SG, Mackenzie AC, Brown CH, *et al.* The Good Behaviour Game and the future of prevention and treatment. *Addict Sci Clin Pract.* 2011; **6**(1): 73.

20 Miller T, Hendrie D. *Substance Abuse Prevention Dollars and Cents: a cost-benefit analysis.* DHHS Pub. No. (SMA) 07–4298. Rockville, MD: Center for Substance Abuse Prevention, Substance Abuse and Mental Health Services Administration; 2009.

21 Conrod PJ, O'Leary-Barrett M, Newton N, *et al.* Effectiveness of a selective, personality-targeted prevention program for adolescent alcohol use and misuse: a cluster randomized controlled trial. *JAMA Psychiatry.* 2013; **70**(3): 334–42.

22 Crome IB, Baldacchino A. The young person's perspective. In: Cooper DB, editor. *Responding in Mental Health: substance use.* London: Radcliffe Publishing; 2011. pp. 48–60.

23 James PD, Smyth, BP. The child's perspective. In: Cooper DB, editor. *Responding in Mental Health – Substance Use.* London: Radcliffe Publishing; 2011. pp. 61–76.

24 European Monitoring Centre for Drugs and Drug Addiction (EMCDDA). *Preventing Later Substance Use Disorders in At-Risk Children and Adolescents: a review of the theory and evidence base of indicated prevention.* Luxembourg: Office for Official Publications of the European Communities; 2009.

25 Hutchings J, Bywater T, Daley D, *et al.* Parenting intervention in Sure Start services for children at risk of developing conduct disorder: pragmatic randomised controlled trial. *BMJ.* 2007; **334**(7595): 678.

26 Anderson P, De Bruijn A, Angus K, *et al.* Impact of alcohol advertising and media exposure on adolescent alcohol use: a systematic review of longitudinal studies. *Alcohol Alcohol.* 2009; **44**(3): 229–43.

CHAPTER 7

What is 'treatment' and who needs it?

INTRODUCTION

Before discussing treatment approaches, it is worth considering the very concept of *treatment*. The word 'treatment' is usually reserved for interventions that are delivered by health professionals to people with diseases. Is substance use a disease? Most people would not view use, per se, as an illness. We view simple use as a behaviour that the person is choosing, albeit a risky behaviour. Interestingly, most Western cultures view alcohol use as an acceptable behaviour, and perceive it as posing low or no risk for young adults.

As discussed in Chapter 2, many risk behaviours have their onset during adolescence. In addition to substance use, these behaviours can include driving too fast, 'bunking off' school, physical fights and unprotected sex. Even where teenagers repeatedly behave this way, we don't view them as having an illness in need of treatment. However, if a young person repeatedly engages in antisocial and risky activities they may get a diagnosis of conduct disorder (*see* Chapter 13). Historically, Western societies have viewed this spectrum of risky behaviours in moral terms, seeing the person as 'bad'. Substance use, like other delinquent behaviour, was met with punishment. Early treatment responses in substance abuse, such as Alcoholics Anonymous (AA) and therapeutic communities (*see* Chapter 11), consequently focused on getting participants to acknowledge the gross errors in their past behaviours.

Substance use could also be compared with behaviours such as deliberate self-harm or self-induced vomiting. These behaviours, which are also choices, are framed in a more sympathetic, health-focused discourse. We view them as maladaptive coping strategies demonstrated by people with mental health or psychological difficulty. Might substance use be the same? It is our assertion that, for some teenagers, it is.

Repeated substance use by teenagers is associated with a broad range of possible adverse consequences for themselves and for those around them. Whether or not one views this behaviour in moral, psychological or mental health terms, there is a need to intervene sometimes. At what point should one seek to intervene? For professionals it can be difficult to identify teenagers with problems and secondly, to know what to do with the problem. This raises challenges for organisations. It evokes three specific issues.

1 *Role legitimacy*: 'Is it *my* job to ask about this teenager's substance use?'
2 *Role adequacy*: 'Do I have the skills to enquire about a teenager's drinking?' 'I don't know enough about drugs, so will the teenager think I'm foolish, asking dumb questions?'
3 *Role support*: 'What will I do if they tell me they are having problems with drug use?' 'There is nowhere to send them if they do need help, so I just won't ask.'

Given the fact that substance use problems are common in adolescence, we believe professionals who work with adolescents should view exploration of substance use as a legitimate part of their role. This is where organisations' policies are extremely important. Staff should be given the competencies to assess and intervene. Unfortunately, many youth services across the world do not have well-developed substance use policies. A culture of 'don't ask and don't tell' can occur. This results in problems being ignored, and means opportunities for early intervention are missed (*see* Box 7.1).

BOX 7.1 Does your organisation assess adolescent substance use?

Is there a drug and/or alcohol use/abuse policy?

Is it clear that all staff should be prepared to talk to adolescents about substance use? If not, is this role delegated to one particular staff member?

Are adolescents automatically asked 'screening questions' about their substance use?

If a teenager has a substance use problem, do you have the skills to work with them? If not, is there someone you can turn to in your organisation or a clear mechanism for accessing external assistance?

If a teenager has a substance use problem, is it clear who must be informed, and in what circumstances (e.g. line manager, the teenager's family, child welfare services)?

Looking at your responses, does your organisation provide a caring environment for adolescents that facilitates problems being identified and responded to supportively?

TERMINOLOGY USED TO DESCRIBE PROBLEMATIC USE OF SUBSTANCES

There are many expressions used to describe substance problems. This can be frustrating! The purpose of this language is to discriminate between different levels of severity. Basically, problems associated with use can be described as low, moderate or severe risk. It is useful to draw distinctions, as the response should be influenced by the problem severity. However, the multitude of terms to describe similar levels of problem can cause confusion. We have summarised some of this terminology in Box 7.2.

BOX 7.2 Terminology used to describe levels of problematic substance use

Problem severity	Terms used to describe
No use	Abstinent, clean, sober
Non-problematic (low-risk) use	Drinking socially; alcohol or drug use*
Moderately problematic use	Substance abuse, substance misuse, substance use disorder, harmful use
Severely problematic use	Substance dependence syndrome, addiction, chemical dependency, drug addict, alcoholism, alcoholic

Note: *This category can be controversial when considering adolescents. Many cultures permit drinking by 16-year-olds. Therefore, the concept of adolescent alcohol use may be uncontentious in those countries. However, few would agree it is reasonable to view a 13-year-old injecting heroin once a month as just heroin use. Such behaviour would be viewed as at least moderately problematic, and therefore warranting significant intervention.

In addition to confusion around language about problem severity, there is significant variation regarding terminology used to discuss specific substances. While most professionals involved in addiction treatment view alcohol as 'just another drug', this is not always the case. Politically, there is reluctance to call alcohol a drug. For this reason, treatment providers may specify that they deal with drugs *and* alcohol. Services may indicate they deal with both by declaring that they work with problematic use of '*substances*', '*chemicals*' or '*psychoactive drugs*'. The expression *illicit drug* abuse is used to describe abuse of drugs that are illegal (such as cannabis). Abuse of *licit drugs* implies use of substances that can be prescribed by doctors (such as benzodiazepines) but may include drugs that are sold legally, such as alcohol.

SCREENING FOR SUBSTANCE USE PROBLEMS

Being unsure what questions to ask can be a reason why adults fail to explore adolescents' substance use. In other words, it is a role-adequacy issue. In order to enquire about substance use, it helps, but is not essential, to have a pre-existing relationship with the adolescent. Prior to asking sensitive questions you should let the teenager know why you are asking them and outline the extent of confidentiality (*see* Chapter 17). It helps if you can come from a position of concern, and ask questions as part of a conversation, as opposed to via a regimented, 'tick box' assessment. You might say something like:

> At this service, we try to get a good understanding about what is going on for those we work with. We want to find out about the things in your life that are going well and the things that could be going better . . . Some young people use drugs and alcohol. I would like to ask you a couple of questions about that, if that is okay?

Try to convey curiosity and avoid verbal or non-verbal responses that may be perceived as judgemental if the adolescent reports substance use. It is helpful to keep opening questions brief and to stay focused upon the more commonly encountered issues. Levy and colleagues[1] recommend three simple questions.

1 Have you drunk alcohol?
   — Give examples of the drinks used by adolescents, such as beer, cider, vodka, as some teenagers think that 'alcohol' only applies to spirits.
2 Have you smoked marijuana, hash or 'weed'?
   — Try to use the terminology relevant to your context, especially if using slang terms such as 'weed'. Other terms may include 'skunk', 'grass', 'blunts', and so forth (*see* Chapter 3).
3 Have you used anything else to get 'high' or for 'a buzz'?

If the answer to these questions is no, the discussion could end there. However, there could still be value in asking teenagers if they were in situations where they could have used. If they were, affirm them for non-use and explore why they opted not to use. This may have value from a prevention perspective, as they explain their decision for *non-use*, which will usually be based upon the perceived negative consequence. This strategy of discussing non-use may build their motivation to continue to avoid future use.

If the adolescent reports use of one or more substances it is necessary to undertake further screening. A useful template for this is the CRAFFT questions developed by the Boston Children's Hospital.[2] The CRAFFT questions are straightforward and do not require the interviewer to have a comprehensive knowledge of substance use (*see* Box 7.3).

BOX 7.3 CRAFFT screening questions

1   Have you ever ridden in a **C**ar driven by someone (including yourself) who
    was high or had been using alcohol or drugs?
2   Do you ever use alcohol or drugs to **R**elax, feel better about yourself, or fit in?
3   Do you ever use alcohol or drugs while you are by yourself **A**lone?
4   Do you ever **F**orget things you did while using alcohol or drugs?
5   Do your **F**amily or **F**riends ever tell you that you should cut down on your
    drinking or drug use?
6   Have you ever gotten into **T**rouble while you were using alcohol or drugs?

Scoring: Two or more positive items indicates the need for further assessment.

There are more-detailed screening instruments available – these might be considered in organisations dealing with larger numbers of substance-using adolescents. Two instruments worthy of consideration are the Global Appraiser of Individual Needs Short Screener (GAIN-SS) or the Alcohol, Smoking and Substance Involvement Screening Test (ASSIST).

The Lighthouse Institute developed the GAIN-SS. It can be self-administered or staff administered, taking 5 minutes to complete. It explores mental health symptoms, antisocial and criminal behaviours and substance use. While not complex, some questions require staff to have a good knowledge of substance use and its attendant problems. While it is available online (www.gaincc.org/GAINSS), services that use it are asked to register with the developers for the cost of US$100 per 5-year period.

The ASSIST was developed for the World Health Organization and is more adult focused than the GAIN-SS. An adolescent version is currently under development. Information can be obtained online (www.who.int/substance_abuse/activities/assist/en/index.html).

RESPONDING TO SUBSTANCE USE PROBLEMS

Adolescent-specific services will inevitably encounter teenagers who have substance use problems. Most countries have developed services tasked specifically with providing interventions for adolescents with more severe problems. Therefore, just as there is a spectrum of problems within any population of adolescents, there is also a spectrum of services that vary in their capacity to respond to problems of increasing complexity. In the UK and Ireland, these services are described according to a four-tier model.[3,4]

Tier 1 includes generic services. Some have a remit to deal with the general adolescent population (e.g. schools) and some deal with adolescents and other age ranges (e.g. doctors, probation officers). While staff working in these services may have highly developed competencies in their area of expertise, their skills in managing adolescent substance use issues are modest, but not non-existent.

Staff working in Tier 2 services have greater ability to assess and intervene in adolescent substance use problems. However, this is not the core focus of their work.

Tier 3 services are specialist multidisciplinary outpatient adolescent substance use services. These treatment services contain professionals with a broad range of competencies relevant to managing adolescents with complex substance use problems. Key competencies existing within the ideal Tier 3 multidisciplinary team include the ability to:

- assess developmental issues
- deliver individual (and/or group) counselling interventions, such as Adolescent Community Reinforcement Approach, cognitive behavioural therapy and group-based cognitive behavioural therapy
- deliver systemic/family therapy
- assess child protection issues
- retain adolescents in treatment
- deliver medical treatment for addiction disorders
- assess and treat co-morbid physical and mental health disorders.

No one individual or profession will have all of the competencies listed here. Therefore, the team will necessarily be multidisciplinary. Internationally, services at Tier 3 are underdeveloped, although this is gradually changing.

Tier 4 services deal with the most complex cases, and offer an intensive therapeutic intervention, which is usually residential. However, services that operate like a day hospital, providing many hours of client contact, may also be considered Tier 4.

Where four tiers exist, it is expected that referrals for treatment will be made by services at Tiers 1 and 2. Following referral, clients will be assessed in the Tier 3 service, which will be capable of meeting the needs of the majority of adolescents. However, where needs are deemed high risk, the Tier 3 team may refer to the Tier 4 service for a period of intensive treatment. The historical absence of Tier 3 services has meant many clients have been referred directly into Tier 4 treatment, where their needs could have been met by a locally delivered and vastly cheaper Tier 3 intervention.

Service provision varies from country to country and often varies by geographic location within countries. We recommend you identify the potential providers of treatment interventions for substance-using adolescents in *your* locality. Clarify the referral criteria of the identified services as follows.

- Is there a specific catchment area that they cover?
- Is there an upper or lower age limit?
- Do they deal with alcohol *and* other drugs?
- Who can and cannot make referrals?
- What is the typical delay between referral and an assessment appointment?
- What treatment model do they use?

Obtaining answers to these questions will save time and make it easier to refer if and when you need to. High-quality and helpful Tier 2, 3 and 4 services should respond to general or specific queries by telephone. If you are unsure about the appropriateness of a referral, a simple phone call may assist you.

In an effort to ensure more rational use of finite treatment resources, the American Society of Addiction Medicine (ASAM) has developed Patient Placement Criteria, which involve assessment of adolescents across six domains of functioning.[5,6] As in the four-tier model, the spectrum of services are ranked by intensity and complexity of the intervention. Table 7.1 outlines this spectrum and indicates the comparable level within the four-tier model.

TABLE 7.1 Categories of treatment service type based upon American Society of Addiction Medicine (ASAM) guidelines

	ASAM PPC-2R level of care	Approximate equivalent in the UK and Irish four-tier model
0.5	Early intervention	Tier 1
I	Outpatient	Tier 2
II	Intensive outpatient and partial hospital	
II.1	Intensive outpatient	Tier 3
II.5	Partial hospital/day programme	
III	Residential/inpatient	
III.1	Clinically managed low-intensity residential	Tier 4
III.5	Clinically managed medium-intensity residential	
III.7	Medically monitored high-intensity residential/ inpatient	
IV	Medically managed, hospital ward-type setting	

Note: PPC, Patient Placement Criteria; adapted from Fishman[7]

Determining patient placement requires considerable knowledge of substance use disorders and coexisting problems. Therefore, it is not usually done by

professionals working in non-addiction services. The main function of the ASAM assessment is to assist in decision-making *within* specialist substance abuse services, especially to discriminate patients requiring residential treatment from those who can be managed in an outpatient treatment. The six domains considered when using the ASAM Patient Placement Criteria are:
1 intoxication and withdrawal potential
2 biomedical conditions and complications
3 emotional, behavioural, and cognitive conditions and complications
4 readiness to change
5 relapse and continued use potential
6 recovery environment.

Detailed discussion regarding these criteria is beyond the scope of this book, but the interested reader can read Mee-Lee.[6]

EMERGENCY TREATMENT
Adolescents with severe substance use problems can encounter points of acute crises in their lives. Suicidal behaviour may be evident; they can accidentally overdose; some may become paranoid or psychotic; they may engage in serious crime while intoxicated, or in efforts to fund drug use; they may engage in prostitution or enter concerning sexual relationships with older substance-using partners; their accommodation placement, whether it is with family or in the care system, may break down because of 'unmanageable' behaviour. These coexisting problems can cause huge distress to parents and wider family. A sense of frustration grows and there may be increasing awareness that 'something must be done'.

At these times, pressure is often put on addiction services, especially residential, to provide immediate responses. However, few residential services respond in this manner. Referrers and the adults involved in the adolescent's life can become angry at this situation. Oftentimes, the family is really looking for respite from the acute problem. The function of treatment services is to provide treatment, not respite. In order to maximise likelihood that treatment has a good outcome, it is good practice to conduct a comprehensive assessment prior to admission. During the pre-admission process, efforts will be undertaken to build the teenagers' motivation to engage in treatment. The adolescents themselves may have little interest in tackling their substance use. As treatment requires their active and sustained participation, it is pointless to enforce admission in an unplanned manner. Referrers may have an expectation that the adolescent can be admitted and that the service will 'make the person want to change'. This rarely happens. While movies may present stories of people undergoing cathartic moments of insight during treatment, it is unreasonable to admit unmotivated, unprepared adolescents into expensive, intensive treatments in the forlorn hope that they discover motivation while in treatment.

Consequently, we share the view that, although teenagers with substantial drug or alcohol problems can frequently encounter emergency situations, there is very rarely a role for emergency entry into addiction treatment to solve these problems.

So, how should crises be handled in the real world? We argue that most of these scenarios require multi-agency involvement, with the addiction service being one such agency. If the issue causing most concern is a mental health issue (i.e. suicidality), then the adolescent mental health service should have a lead role until that acute problem has abated. If there are accommodation or child protection issues, then child welfare services should take the lead role, with input from addiction services. These are complex problems that require complex solutions. No one service can solve all the issues for adolescents. While the notion that a very high-risk teenager's life can be sorted by a 6-week addiction treatment admission alone is an attractive one, it is rarely borne out by reality. Typically, many challenges such adolescents face in their lives predate their substance use. Therefore it is folly to expect cessation of their substance use will normalise their lives. It is important that we do not build unrealistic expectations of the addiction service. Excellent outcomes can occur, but they are relatively uncommon. Where they occur, they usually have their origins in solid, planned and organised inter-agency work, in collaboration with active families.

DIAGNOSING ADOLESCENTS WHO HAVE SUBSTANCE USE PROBLEMS

People who demonstrate certain groups of symptoms are said to have a specific diagnosis. It is helpful for health professionals to have a shared understanding regarding each illness they encounter. This is the case across all medical specialties. For example, endocrinologists working in Australia use the same diagnostic criteria for insulin-dependent diabetes as those used in the United States. If this were not the case, then it would be impossible for doctors in Australia to interpret the results of research studies conducted by colleagues in the United States. Medical diagnoses of physical illnesses have advanced greatly in the last century and there is now good understanding of the origins of most illnesses. There are medical investigations (such as blood tests) that allow additional objectivity to diagnostic categories rather than simply relying on physical examinations or patient-reported symptoms.

Unfortunately, in the area of mental health, there is less certainty. Most diagnoses are based on patient report of a range of symptoms. Nevertheless, it is equally important that clinicians worldwide share an understanding of the disorders they treat. Therefore, psychiatrists working in Africa use the same diagnostic criteria to determine if a patient has schizophrenia as their colleagues in Britain. As research advances, diagnostic criteria are reviewed and modified accordingly.

The World Health Organization has produced guidelines on diagnostic criteria for diseases called the International Classification of Diseases (ICD). These guidelines are reviewed intermittently. The current criteria, ICD-10, were agreed in 1992. The ICD-10 uses the term *dependence syndrome* to explain addiction. It is stated, 'the central descriptive characteristic of the dependence syndrome is the desire to take psychoactive drugs'.[8] They list a number of key diagnostic criteria. There must be at least three of these in the past year for a person to be diagnosed with a *dependence syndrome*. The core symptoms are:

- a strong desire or compulsion to take the substance (e.g. cravings)
- difficulties in controlling substance-taking behaviour (e.g. if the person starts using on a night out, they often have difficulty stopping or limiting their use)
- physiological withdrawal (e.g. 'cold turkey' symptoms occur when they stop heroin use)
- evidence of tolerance (i.e. the person needs more of the substance to get the same effect)
- neglect of alternative pleasures or interest because of substance use (increasing time is spent obtaining, using or recovering from the substance, and alternative aspects of life are progressively neglected)
- persisting with use despite clear evidence of harmful consequences (e.g. the person can see that the substance use has a negative impact on his or her mental health but continues to use).[8]

These diagnostic criteria were developed with adults in mind. However, the same criteria are used for adolescents. There are some issues worth noting when considering the appropriateness of these diagnostic criteria for adolescents. First, withdrawal symptoms are relatively uncommon in teenagers. We tend to see a pattern of heavy *episodic* use of substances in adolescents. However, physical dependence typically requires the substance user to engage in a sustained period of *daily* use. Secondly, in Anglo-Saxon cultures, drinkers often use alcohol to the point of intoxication. On commencement of drinking, people typically notice that their tolerance to alcohol rises over that first year. However, using ICD-10 criteria, tolerance constitutes one of the features of dependence.

The other diagnostic category within ICD-10 is *harmful use*. This specifies that the pattern of substance use has caused damage to either physical or mental health. Adverse social consequences such as school problems or criminal charges do *not* constitute harmful use according to ICD-10 criteria. Physical health problems associated with regular substance use are relatively uncommon in adolescents. Mental health symptoms commonly coexist with regular substance use in adolescents, but the diagnosis of harmful use can only be made where these symptoms can be confidently attributed to the substance use.

The alternative diagnostic criteria are the the Diagnostic and Statistical Manual of Mental Disorders (DSM), known as DSM-IV-TR, categories, which have been determined by the American Psychiatric Association. Overall, their diagnostic criteria are similar to the ICD-10. Up until 2013 in DSM-IV they also used two categories. Firstly, there was *substance dependence*, and the diagnostic criteria were almost identical to the ICD-10 *dependence syndrome* outlined earlier. The less-severe category in DSM-IV was called *substance abuse*. It was a wider category than the harmful use diagnosis used in ICD-10. A person, whether adult or adolescent, could be diagnosed with substance abuse if they encountered social problems or engaged in criminal activity linked to their substance use.

The DSM criteria were updated in 2013. The two diagnostic categories have been merged and they opted to cease use of the words 'abuse' and 'dependence', which are perceived to be pejorative. There is a single category called *substance use disorders*, which are subcategorised as mild, moderate or severe, depending upon the number of symptoms identified.

THE DISEASE MODEL

Historically, there was a belief that addiction was a disease. The history of this model is outlined in Box 7.4. Most writings on the disease model have focused on alcohol. Most people drink alcohol and the majority can use it without it causing major harm. However, a minority of drinkers seem unable to use alcohol in a controlled or moderate manner. There was a view that such 'alcoholics' had a disease and the fact that they had this disease meant they were simply unable to drink alcohol in a non-damaging manner. Ongoing drinking would inevitably lead to an inexorable physical, psychological and moral decline. Organisations such as AA embrace this disease model. The afflicted individual has to cease alcohol use forever, and the 12 steps of AA provide the (only) path to an escape. It presents a very 'all or nothing' view of addiction, and lifelong abstinence as the *only* solution.

While the diagnostic criteria outlined in ICD-10 and DSM-IV seek to define the illness of addiction or dependence, they do not rigidly subscribe to the view that it is an 'all or nothing' disease. DSM V has more clearly moved towards the view that substance use disorders are a broad spectrum. This is important for adolescents. Substance use can escalate rapidly during adolescence driven by a range of factors including the context in which the teenager lives and an under-developed repertoire of coping skills. Adolescents can go down some unhelpful behavioural 'cul de sacs', such as substance use. As their context changes and their social skills develop, they can make major changes. Therefore, we do not subscribe to the disease model as *the* cause of all addiction. While there may well be individual teenagers who have a 'disease' which means they can never reasonably hope to revert to low-risk use, we cannot currently distinguish such individuals from the other teenagers who also meet the diagnostic criteria for dependence but who can and do achieve major behavioural change without lifelong abstinence.

Some challenges to the disease model include the following points.

- Decades ago it emerged that some people attained controlled drinking at follow-up despite a history of severe alcohol dependence.[9]
- The evidence that context is a major influence on addictive behaviour comes as a challenge to the disease model. The power of context was most impressively demonstrated in studies of heroin dependence in Vietnam vets in the 1970s.[10] While in the stressful war environment, with access to cheap high-quality heroin, and surrounded by heroin-abusing comrades, many soldiers became heroin dependent. However, lots of these soldiers immediately and permanently ceased heroin use with ease upon their return to the United States.

Interestingly, although the disease model is falling out of favour, the view that addiction is a brain disease is being proposed with increasing vigour by organisations such as the National Institute on Drug Abuse in the United States. This theory has its origins in the ever-increasing evidence of abnormalities in brain functioning seen in people with histories of regular substance use. Importantly, the differences in functioning between people *with* and *without* addictions are only evident when you look at the *average* findings across the two groups. There is overlap in brain functioning between people with and without addictions and therefore there is no 'cut-off' or biological test to reliably identify people with addictions.

BOX 7.4 A history and background to the disease model of addiction

The idea that addiction is a disease is not a new one. In the book *Slaying the Dragon*,[11] we are told 'the birth of the American Disease Concept' started with Dr Benjamin Rush. He presented 'the first fully formed conception of alcohol addiction as a disease'.[12] Rush proposed that 'once an appetite or "craving" for spirits had developed, the victim was powerless to resist'.[12]

More recently, Professor David Clark[13] informed us that the 'heart of this [the disease] model is that addiction is characterised by a person's inability to reliably control his use of alcohol or drugs and an uncontrollable craving or compulsion to drink or take drugs.' However, the cause of addiction is explained differently by different disease models.[13] Heathers and Robertson[12] suggest there are three main disease models.

Pre-existent physical abnormality

This approach supports genetic factors. In this model, the addict is seen as possessing some 'biochemical abnormality which leads him to react differently to the substance from all other human beings and which causes addiction'.[12]

Addiction as a mental illness or psychopathology

This suggests that addiction is a mental illness, that the predisposition is not a physical one, but rather 'a psychological abnormality'.[12]

Acquired addiction or dependence

This is the most common disease model. What makes this model different is the fact that 'the disease the alcoholic suffers from does not precede his drinking but is a consequence of it' (i.e. the alcohol itself causes the disease).[12]

Terrance Gorski[14] states, 'to intelligently discuss the issue of whether or not alcoholism is a disease, we must first define disease.' He contests that alcohol dependence affects the brain and does damage to other organ systems and that there are clear, identifiable groups of signs and symptoms, which is arguably true, as both the ICD-10 and the DSM-IV give a list of symptoms for alcohol and drug dependence.[14]

ADOLESCENT TREATMENT PROGRAMMES

Adolescents constitute a small proportion of the overall population of people with severe substance problems. The treatment programmes for addiction have almost all been developed for adults. As the number of adolescents with problems has escalated, there have been efforts to develop adolescent-specific treatment programmes. In most cases, this has meant adapting the adult models of treatment, to make them more developmentally appropriate.

There are a number of ways in which adolescents with addiction issues differ from adults (*see* Box 7.5). Services that are adapting an adult model of treatment need to address each of these when making adaptions.

BOX 7.5 Issues which differentiate substance-using adolescents from substance-using adults

Greater reliance upon family

Adolescents are more reliant upon their family. Consequently, they do better in treatment when parents are involved. Some families struggle to provide the ideal level of support and this can compromise outcome. Involving parents in treatment poses a challenge to some models of treatment that typically focus more upon the individual client. There can be challenges in terms of confidentiality and consent.

Less ability to change their social context and exit unhealthy relationships

Adolescents have less ability than adults to move away from neighbourhoods where drug use is endemic. They also have less ability to distance themselves from unhealthy loving relationships (i.e. a 14-year-old cannot end his or her relationship with his or her alcohol-dependent mother, but a 34-year-old can).

Greater focus on education

Treatment services need to establish an understanding of and links with the education system when working with adolescents.

More likely to be on an upward trajectory in their substance use

Substance use waxes and wanes over life. Adults are more likely to enter treatment when things are at their worst. Adolescents may enter treatment when *other* people get concerned. This may be early in the substance use 'career' and occur while problems are on an upward trajectory. In such situations, an intervention which simply halts this escalation in problems may be viewed as useful.

Motivation is poorer

Adults typically seek treatment themselves. Adolescents are generally referred by others. Therefore, their motivation to enter treatment and make changes is poorer than adults, on average.

Less likely to have chronic physical health problems

The chronic health problems associated with substance use tend to be related to accumulated lifetime use. Such problems are relatively uncommon in adolescents.

Present with child welfare issues

Adult services encounter dilemmas regarding child protection concerns that arise from the parenting of the children of their clients. Different but equally complex challenges arise for the clients of adolescent services, as these are legally identified as children themselves.

Focus is on habilitation, not rehabilitation

The word 'rehabilitation' implies efforts to restore a *pre-existing* level of functioning. This can be done for a 30-year-old with a 5-year history of cocaine dependence. This person can rediscover the lifestyle and coping skills of their early twenties. However, a fundamentally different approach is required for a 16-year-old. There will not be a goal of restoring them to the functioning of their 12-year-old pre-addicted self. The goals must be to give them skills and to guide them towards a lifestyle they have never previously had. This is more challenging than simply rehabilitation.

With these issues in mind, Brannigan and colleagues[15] identified 45 key ingredients of the ideal specialist adolescent addiction programme. These key ingredients were grouped into nine areas (*see* Box 7.6). They then assessed the 144 most highly regarded adolescent treatment services in the United States to measure their adherence to these ideal standards. Across these services the median score was 23 out of 45 elements. They found 'the elements with the poorest-quality performance were assessment and treatment matching, engaging and retaining teens in treatment, gender and cultural competence, and [measurement of] treatment outcomes'. One component of assessment that was frequently lacking was mental health. In view of common mental health co-morbidities, it is important that adolescent services have the competence to assess and manage the most common mental health problems.

BOX 7.6 Key elements of effective adolescent drug treatment programmes[15]

1   *Assessment and treatment matching*: programmes should conduct comprehensive assessments that cover psychiatric, psychological and medical problems, learning disabilities, family functioning, and other aspects of the adolescent's life.
2   *Comprehensive, integrated treatment approach*: programmes should address all aspects of an adolescent's life.
3   *Family involvement in treatment*: involving parents in the adolescent's treatment produces better outcomes.

(Continued)

BOX 7.6 (cont.)

4 *Developmentally appropriate programme:* activities and materials should reflect the developmental differences between adults and adolescents.

5 *Engaging and retaining teens in treatment:* programmes should build a climate of trust between adolescents and therapists.

6 *Qualified staff:* staff should be trained in adolescent development, mental disorders and substance use.

7 *Gender and cultural competence:* programmes should address the distinct needs of adolescent boys and girls, as well as cultural differences among minorities.

8 *Continuing care:* programmes should include relapse prevention training, aftercare plans, referrals to community resources and follow-up.

9 *Treatment outcomes:* rigorous evaluation is required to measure success, target resources and improve treatment services.

TREATMENT OUTCOMES

Treatment outcomes in adolescent substance abuse are modest. Even in situations where teenagers fully adhere to a treatment programme, many fail to attain good outcomes. This is the case across all treatment modalities, and comparisons across different treatments yield similar results. There is good evidence that adolescents do better in treatment interventions that involve family, such as Multidimensional Family Therapy.[16] Nevertheless, it is only about one-quarter of patients who achieve good outcomes following treatment. A further 50% achieve modest improvements. The remaining one-quarter show no benefit. Importantly, teenagers who do badly following one particular treatment episode may have an excellent outcome if they re-enter treatment later, even if it is back into the same treatment model that did not work previously.

It is also important to consider what constitutes a good outcome. The public tend to have an expectation that a good outcome means an adolescent ceases substance use forever. This view may be influenced by the dominance of the disease model concept among the general population. This perfect outcome is extremely difficult to attain. Generally, outcome studies look 3–12 months after the treatment interventions and generate the outcomes mentioned above. Therefore, setting lifelong abstinence as the benchmark for 'good outcome' is probably unrealistic for both treatment services and the clients who access them.

Irrespective of treatment modality, treatment retention is another predictor of treatment outcome. People who stick with treatment do better.

Consequently, many treatment models developed recently place great emphasis on ensuring treatment is delivered in a patient-centred, collaborative and
flexible manner. Historically, services viewed treatment dropout as a failure by
the client, indicating that they were not ready or were in denial. More recently
and maybe influenced by therapies such as Motivational Interviewing, *dropout
is viewed as a service failure*, not a client failure.

Treatment services generally ask adolescents, their families and referrers to
look broadly when considering outcomes. Most good interventions will explore
many aspects of the adolescent's functioning including mental health, their
ability to form meaningful relationships, participation in criminal activity,
and progression in terms of vocational or educational attainment. Therefore,
treatment services will often view an outcome as 'good' if a person makes a
substantial improvement in two or three of these domains, even if some substance use persists.

Over the past 2 decades, there has been an increase in the number of services
that offer 'harm reduction interventions'. These services do not insist on abstinence as a necessary goal for the patient to have upon treatment entry. However,
it is a goal that a person can certainly be encouraged to work towards. Harm
reduction interventions permit the adolescent to set goals of reducing use and
to tackle coexisting problems that are present in their lives as a result of their
use, while postponing any final decision regarding abstinence. Treatment interventions such as Motivational Interviewing and the Adolescent Community
Reinforcement Approach adopt this latter harm reduction approach and are
described in subsequent chapters. Treatment interventions that insist on abstinence include 12-step programmes and therapeutic communities described in
Chapter 11.

Is it realistic to expect all adolescents to obtain abstinence? Alternatively, are
some teenagers being 'sold short' by being offered harm reduction programmes
as opposed to insisting that they cease all substance abuse? It is interesting to
look to other areas within the health arena when contemplating these questions. Obviously, lifelong abstinence constitutes the perfect outcome. However,
throughout all aspects of healthcare, professionals find themselves increasingly managing chronic conditions that run an intermittent, fluctuating and
relapsing course. Symptoms oscillate over time and treatment is typically episodic throughout life. In reality, when we look at patients with the spectrum
of substance use problems, especially those at the severe end, we notice they
run a similar chronic and relapsing course. Therefore it is unrealistic to expect
that everyone will attain abstinence. However, it is also a fact that some people, even those with the most severe, entrenched addictions, do occasionally
move to this perfect outcome. It is vital that these rare and spectacular 'recov-
eries' do not build unrealistic expectations about treatment or similarly cause

us to berate services that fail to regularly deliver such remarkable outcomes. It is generally accepted that a patient who has multiple severe morbidities such as chronic obstructive airways disease, lung cancer and congestive heart failure is going to have a modest outcome despite high-quality and world-class treatment. Unfortunately, in the sphere of mental health there continues to be unrealistic expectations that patients with multiple severe morbidities such as severe cocaine dependence, an emotionally unstable personality disorder and bipolar affective disorder would have a great outcome if they could 'only find the right doctor or the right treatment'.

CONCLUSION AND KEY POINTS

- As substance use is common in adolescents, services that work with teenagers should ensure that substance use is screened for.
- Staff require training in screening and early interventions.
- Adolescents are different to adults and they require different treatment approaches. Family involvement is important.
- International diagnostic criteria such as ICD-10 and DSM-V, while imperfect and subject to review, ensure greater uniformity in categorisation of problems across the world.
- There should be a range of treatment responses for adolescents with substance use problems, with the intensity of the response matched to the severity of the substance use disorder.

REFERENCES

1 Levy S, Winters KC, Knight J. Screening, assessment and triage for treatment at a primary care setting. In: Kaminer Y, Winters KC, editors. *Clinical Manual Of Adolescent Substance Abuse Treatment.* Washington, DC: American Psychiatric Association; 2011. pp. 65–82.

2 Knight JR, Sherritt L, Shrier LA, *et al.* Validity of the CRAFFT substance abuse screening test among adolescent clinic patients. *Arch Pediatr Adolesc.* 2002; **156**(6): 607–14.

3 Department of Health and Children. *Report of the Working Group on Treatment of Under 18s Presenting to Treatment Services with Serious Drug Problems.* Dublin: Department of Health and Children; 2005.

4 Health Advisory Service. *Substance of Young Need.* London: Health Advisory Service; 2001.

5 American Society of Addiction Medicine (ASAM). *Patient Placement Criteria-2R [PPC-2R].* Chevy Chase, MD: ASAM; 2007.

6 Mee-Lee D. *The Revised Second Edition ASAM Patient Placement Criteria: understanding and using ASAM PPC-2R.* Davis, CA. 2009. Available at: www.samhsa.gov/co-occurring/

topics/screening-and-assessment/ASAMPatientPlacementCriteriaOverview5-05.pdf (accessed 9 August 2013).

7 Fishman M. Placement criteria and treatment planning for adolescents with substance use disorders. In: Kaminer Y, Winters KC, editors. *Clinical Manual of Adolescent Substance Abuse Treatment.* Washington, DC: American Psychiatric Association; 2011. pp. 113–42.

8 World Health Organization (WHO). *The ICD-10 Classification of Mental and Behavioural Disorders.* Geneva: WHO; 1992.

9 Davies DL. Normal drinking in recovered alcohol addicts. *Q J Stud Alcohol.* 1962; **23**: 94–104.

10 Robins LN. Vietnam veterans' rapid recovery from heroin addiction: a fluke or normal expectation? *Addiction.* 1993; **88**(8): 1041–54.

11 White WL. *Slaying the Dragon: the history of addiction treatment and recovery in America.* Bloomington, IL: Chestnut Health Systems Publications; 1998.

12 Heathers N, Robertson I. *Problem Drinking.* 3rd ed. Oxford: Oxford Medical Publications; 1997.

13 Clark D. The disease model of addiction. *Drink Drug News.* 2006; **25**: 15.

14 Gorski T. The disease model of addiction. Paper presented at *The 10th Annual Dual Disorder Conference.* 1996 October 4; Las Vegas, NE. Available at: www.tgorski.com/gorski_articles/disease_model_of_addiction_010704.htm (accessed 16 January 2013).

15 Brannigan R, Schackman BR, Falco M., *et al.* The quality of highly regarded adolescent substance abuse treatment programs: results of an in-depth national survey. *Arch Pediatr Adolesc Med.* 2004; **158**(9): 904–9.

16 Tanner-Smith EE, Wilson SJ, Lipsey MW. The comparative effectiveness of outpatient treatment for adolescent substance abuse: a meta-analysis. *J Subst Abuse Treat.* 2013; **44**(2): 145–58.

CHAPTER 8

Harnessing the significant influence of parents

INTRODUCTION

The use of drugs and alcohol is often central to serious disagreements between parents and teenagers. Frequently, teens see no problem with using illicit substances. Parents become very distressed about this and the effects of substance misuse. Unfortunately, often the teenager does not accept that his or her problems are connected to drug misuse, raising parents' concerns even further. Parents are the ones most likely to notice problems, intervene and insist that the young person makes changes. They can become overwhelmed and hopeless in the face of continuing difficulties. Conflict in the home may persist for many months, even years. Parents may believe they have no positive influence and often feel that they have 'failed'.

Practitioners can support parents to notice achievements in their child-rearing, regain confidence as parents and help them rebuild relationships with their adolescents, re-establishing their desired boundaries and reclaiming peaceful lives. This chapter presents the difficulties faced by parents and ways of working to support them to bring about change in adolescent substance misuse. A brief overview of systemic therapy and narrative approaches to adolescent drug and alcohol misuse are offered. Research-evidenced responses that include parents, carers and family are outlined. If there is uncertainty about which approach to suggest, the wisdom of the parent can provide direction as to what might best fit their situation.

An adolescent may not always be in the care of a parent. The information offered in this chapter can be usefully applied in the context of foster-parents, childcare situations or for whoever is the caregiver of the adolescent, while also holding an awareness of the increased needs of the adolescent and family in those situations.

POLICY AND RESEARCH

The National Drug Strategy in the UK identified the specific needs of family members who are dealing with drug misuse in the home.[1] In 2008 the National Treatment Agency for Substance Misuse in the UK published its guide to ways services can support and involve carers, including them in their family members' drug treatment.[2] Research confirms that involving family members in the treatment of drug misuse problems improves outcomes, particularly in the treatment of adolescent drug misuse.[2-5] In a European survey of teenagers' attitudes towards their substance use, many participants said their parents' opinion mattered. One 17-year-old girl from the Netherlands said:

> If my parents found out I had used ecstasy, my whole life would be messed up, they would never speak to me again. It would be impossible to have a normal relationship with them.[6]

PROBLEMS ENCOUNTERED BY PARENTS

Parents face challenges in managing substance misuse behaviours, which become more concerning as use increases. In an Australian study from 2007, parents found it difficult to live with suspicion, shame, blame and guilt. They named the challenge of trying to keep their teen safe. They described the grief they felt as they let go of their hopes and dreams for their child. They named the sense of having to protect themselves from burnout in trying to cope with the situation.[7] An exploration of problems parents face and possible solutions follows.

Loss of trust

Loss of trust can stem simply from a teen repeatedly promising to be in on time and constantly breaking his or her word. Often the teenager can have good intentions but be carried along with whatever friends are doing or at times deliberately break his or her parents' rules. A teenager may steal money or property from family members to pay for alcohol or drugs. When this is accompanied by denial, it causes confusion, frustration and anger. The problem can escalate to involve significant sums. Parents can take steps to reduce this by being vigilant about money at all times. This can be frustrating but is a containing response from the parent, while the problem persists.

Teenagers sometimes underestimate how difficult it is to regain trust, leading parents to think that the teenager is not taking responsibility for his or her behaviour.

Problems with limit-setting

Adolescent substance use occurs at a time when a teenager ought to be getting increased freedoms. One of the main tasks of adolescence is individuation, when the adolescent requires less protection from parents and begins to take on adult responsibilities (*see* Chapter 4). When the teen requests more freedom while the parent, aware of the teen's substance misuse, believes he or she is not managing freedom well, guidance and consequences are needed.

Often consequences for misdemeanours are seen as punishments. Practitioners can help parents see consequences as messages for the teen rather than punishments. These messages need to be consistent and appropriate. Parents often find the consequences they put in place are ineffective. They report that grounding 'just doesn't work' – the teen walks out. Grounding for one or two evenings is more likely to be implementable than grounding for 2 weeks. This allows the parent to repeat the message that certain behaviour is unacceptable. In reality it is often the drip effect of a persistently repeated message that eventually hits home. Supporting parents to maintain a caring relationship in the midst of ongoing conflict, while continuing to set limits, will benefit both parents and adolescent.

Substance use exists on a continuum. Parents often view drug use in black-and-white terms: using or not using. So when their child reduces from five cannabis joints a day to just one (a reduction of 80%) the improvement isn't noticed. Naturally, this can lead to parents becoming disheartened and teens frustrated. Living with teenagers who are involved with substance use is hard work. Supporting parents to persist in the everyday practices of boundary setting can help.

Differences in parenting approaches

Parents do not always agree when it comes to expectations they have of their children. Many couples will have worked out these differences over the years. However, demands on the couple increase as concerns grow. Adolescents have had years of learning what differences of opinion exist between their parents, and may exploit these. Couples can find that the focus is on their different approaches rather than the actions of their teenager. Finding time to discuss dilemmas and avoiding blaming the other will help. Parents can agree not to disagree in front of the teen.

Relationship breakdown

Ensuring a unified approach becomes even more important when parents separate. Feelings of anger, hurt and guilt often come with separation and can interfere with decision-making. Practitioners can help parents to focus on their parenting role and see that while their couple relationship is ending, their parenting is a lifelong endeavour. Taking time to explore shared values around parenting can help to move conversations to points of agreement.

When parents are not living together it can become tempting to send the child to the other parent when disagreements arise. Although this may provide respite, conflicts can be sidelined rather than worked through. A teen may experience rejection and believe that his or her parent is not able to cope with him or her, placing further strain on the relationship. Teens will benefit if the adults can provide a strong and steady response to challenging behaviour.

Lone parents

Lone parents will naturally face greater challenges, as they are dealing with difficulties single-handedly. Recruiting help from extended family lightens the burden and increases positive involvement with adults other than the parent. Even if there has not been regular contact with family members, when presented with a request, many are willing to help. Small additional supports can create an influence that changes the direction of the teen's life. The importance of self-care for lone parents cannot be overstated.

Disrupted couple relationship

Parents can feel that they are constantly in the eye of the storm as they try to manage adolescent substance misuse. They can be encouraged to give attention to ensuring they care for their couple relationship. Parents often become exhausted; taking a break, when possible, can bring benefits. This may create a dilemma, as leaving a drug-using teen without supervision is not recommended. Recruiting support from extended family is encouraged. Parents often have not confided in family members and are carrying this burden alone. It can bring relief to share their concerns.

Living with shame and blame

Stigma around substance use can have a silencing impact. Many parents find that they want to protect their teen's reputation within the wider family, hoping the difficulties will subside. They may feel embarrassed as they perceive their child's problems are a sign of poor parenting. Many have postponed asking for support, hoping it won't be necessary. Assisting a parent to work through the pros and cons of whatever position they have chosen will help identify what is useful, what they would like to change, and what they need.

Supporting parents to maintain hope helps parents to stay focused in their attempts to support their child. Most teenagers who use substances eventually grow out of it and become competent young adults. Parents usually have more reason to be positive than negative. However, this positive outcome is not guaranteed. Their goal is therefore to help their child to navigate this difficult period as safely and quickly as possible.

Impact of drug debts and threats

One of the major concerns with drug use involves drug holding, carrying or selling. Some teenagers realise that by helping their friends access drugs, they gain credit for themselves to buy drugs. The adolescent often does not see this as dealing. Over time this drug selling increases and many teenagers encounter problems, often ending up in debt. The home, siblings and parents can become the target of threats and/or violence. At this level, police need to be involved. However, these are difficult decisions to make. Some families borrow large sums to repay debts and try to avoid the juvenile justice system. The concerning fact is that paying debts for teens serves to increase their credit worthiness with the drug supplier, continuing the cycle. Talking to community policing services will usually help parents ascertain the level of risk for their child.

Involvement in the juvenile justice system

Many teenage drug users come into conflict with the law, often being brought home by police, receiving informal cautions, being sent to police diversion programmes, receiving juvenile liaison citations and court appearances. Teens may be unconcerned with the consequences of their actions. Many parents' immediate instinct is to protect their child from the juvenile justice system. This is problematic; it can give the message that the parent will help the teen avoid the consequences of breaking the law. Parents can try to see the criminal justice system as allies who can help divert their teen away from criminality. Involvement with the criminal justice system can be a strong motivator for change.

Becoming disheartened, losing hope and self–care

Parents can be invited to pay careful attention to their energy and stress levels. How has the current situation affected the parents' day-to-day life? Often when we are under pressure we neglect activities that create energy, such as eating well, resting and exercising. Practitioners can help parents to reflect on ways they can sustain themselves in the face of challenges. Ask parents to imagine what they might be doing if they weren't dealing with the current difficulties. Can they do some of those activities within existing constraints?

Concerns about their other children

In dealing with a teen's substance use, everyone living in the home is affected. Parents are rightly concerned about the negative effects of arguments, threats, police calling to the home and the presence of drugs on all their family. Parents face the challenge of showing compassion to their teenager while at the same time not giving the impression to other children that substance use is being accepted.

SYSTEMIC APPROACH TO SUPPORTING PARENTS

The behaviour of one family member affects others. If an adolescent does not want to stop substance use, parents can adapt their approach in ways that can prompt change. Some parents feel that the onus is solely on the teenager to change and they should 'just stop using drugs'. However, taking a systemic view, change can begin anywhere in the system. Parents can influence change and take steps to exert their values in their home. Remaining positive is important: if a parent is constantly critical of their teen's drug use, the teen may spend more time with friends as a way of avoiding criticism. While it is important to let teenagers know their behaviour is unacceptable, more time with drug-using friends is counterproductive. Using a systemic perspective, parents can consider whether their approach is getting the desired result.

Systemic theory has evolved over time, reflecting changes in society. While new models have evolved, there is strong rationale for combining the earlier interventionist styles with more recent collaborative approaches.[8] Structural and strategic models from the 1960s are relevant for families dealing with adolescent substance misuse. Structural family therapy looks at who is in charge, the nature of boundaries and triangulated relationships. Strategic Family Therapy notes patterns of behaviour, examines their function, and seeks to help parents disrupt unhelpful patterns by experimenting with alternative responses. The adolescent may approach one parent repeatedly for permissions and gain freedoms that subsequently prove detrimental. This pattern can be disrupted by the other parent taking a more proactive role. Solution-focused approaches invite a collaborative stance that elicit the families' own solutions.

These ways of working include giving attention to the impact of the practitioner on the system. The family's understandings of the situation are paramount. Dallos and Urry[8] suggest that 'looking for patterns', the impact of 'our own personal views' and the influence of 'the wider cultural context' are all necessary in supporting families to create the changes they desire. There is extensive research that confirms that working with parents in formal treatment of adolescent substance misuse problems brings positive and lasting outcomes.[4]

OVERVIEW OF NARRATIVE APPROACH

From a narrative perspective, life is seen as multistoried and these stories are multilayered. Narrative approaches understand that there are dominant stories that stand out in our lives. Dominant stories are those we choose to tell about ourselves, they are stories that frame our lives, the ones through which we understand ourselves and invite others to know us. Narrative approach invites us to dig deeper; to excavate for strength, stories that may have been covered by dominant negative stories.

> It is through stories that we are able to gain a sense of the unfolding of the events of our lives through recent history, and it appears that this sense is vital to the perception of a 'future' that is in any way different from a 'present'.[9]

One may have been the class clown in school. This story may cause other stories to be overlooked. It may be that the story of managing sadness as a result of bereavement has become covered over by the dominant story of being the joker. Using a narrative approach, a practitioner can delve into the powerful stories of parents managing substance misuse. In this journey of peeling back layers of stories, parents are invited to apply skills used in the past, when coping with difficulties, to current challenges.

The forgotten stories are often the stories of strength and commitment in dealing with substance misuse. Stories of repeatedly setting boundaries and applying consequences, only to find that their teen sidesteps them yet again. Stories of trying different ways to engage in conversation with a reluctant teen. Stories of hours searching for a missing young person. Stories of continuing to hope, even when change does not come. There is power in hope; it causes parents to persist in their care, even though they may see no progress. The efforts that parents are making can become invisible, even to themselves, especially if there is little change in their teen's behaviour.

Parents can be helped to step into a place where they see the problem as separate from themselves or their adolescent. Narrative practice, using 'externalising' questions, sees the problem as the problem, not the person as the problem.[10] By externalising problems, parents obtain a different view of their situation which invites creativity and increased possibilities.

Externalising the problem

Parents dealing with adolescent substance misuse often struggle with shame. Narrative work allows us to separate from the experience of shame so that we can see its influence on us, and equally identify times when it has less influence. Noting times when there was power over the feeling of shame can help us make choices about the next steps in relation to it.

The externalising conversation, which has four steps, moves us from a position of naming the problem to stepping into meaning making in our lives.[10] All our actions are founded on beliefs. We feel strongly about particular things because we have beliefs and values that underpin the positions we take towards those issues. A parent can make this externalising journey from reaction to drug misuse, to identifying why they are taking the positions they are taking, to naming the importance of taking those positions. This frees them up to decide which actions are important to them and prompt them to take more of those actions.

Step 1: Naming the problem

Invite the parent to identify what aspect of dealing with his or her adolescent's drug use is most burdensome. Ask the following externalising questions.

- Can you tell me a bit about the problem?
- Can you give it a name? Being clear about the problem breaks it down into manageable parts.
- When did they first notice the problem?
- Do we have the right name for the problem, or do you want to pick a different name?

Step 2: Noting the effects of the problem

Invite the parent to identify the effects of the problem. This deepens the description of the problem and so extends awareness.

- What does the problem get you to do?
- How does the problem get in the way of everyday life?
- What relationships are affected by the problem?
- Are there times when the problem shows up more than others?

Step 3: Taking a position with regard to the problem

Ask the parent to reflect on how they have taken a position in response to the problem. If they feel that they haven't taken a position up to now, what position would they like to take? Help them to identify this. Here we are moving from the world of the problem to the world of parental values.

- Tell me some of the ways you have objected to the problem.
- Are there times you saw that you made a difference to the problem?
- What steps did you take that helped you to make that difference?
- Can you name other ways you hope or plan to reduce this problem?

This leads to the last aspect of externalising the problem where the parent is invited to reflect on the values that inform the position that they have taken. When we think about what is important to us we begin to make sense of our objections to certain activities. This provides clarity about the journey the parent is on, a way of seeing what values underpin their actions and hence encouragement to take further actions.

Step 4: Identifying the importance of taking this position

- What does it say about you as a parent that you are taking these actions?
- What does it say about your hopes for your life and your adolescent's life?
- Why are you refusing to go along with the things the problem brings into your life?
- What is it like to answer these questions?

As the relationship is built with a parent, this externalising journey can be revisited. Instead of being overwhelmed by the intensity of dealing with a teen's substance misuse, parents can see the problem from other perspectives and create solutions through narrative conversations.

EVIDENCE-BASED MODELS

Several research-evidenced models intentionally involve parents when dealing with adolescent substance misuse. It is useful for practitioners to note the parenting component of these. Adolescent Community Reinforcement Approach (ACRA)[11] is presented in Chapter 10. Elements for parents are outlined here.

Although the Non-Violent Resistance (NVR) model was not developed specifically for adolescent substance misuse, it provides a possible response to challenging behaviours that often accompany drug and alcohol misuse.[12-14]

Adolescent Community Reinforcement Approach

The goals of the ACRA are:
- abstinence or reduction of teen substance use
- increase the young person's engagement in prosocial activities
- development of healthy relationships with family and peers.[11]

While most of the work in the ACRA model is completed with the adolescent, there are specific sessions with parents. ACRA recognises that parents have a major influence on their children; therefore, changes in their behaviour can bring about significant changes in the teenager. ACRA encourages parents to focus on ways they can support their child to become involved in healthy, prosocial, non-drug-related activities, while allowing them to feel the natural negative effects of their substance use. The ACRA model outlines three separate sessions that are carried out with parents. The first two sessions are completed with the parents alone and the third with the adolescent and parents together. The sessions happen in parallel with the adolescent engaging in the one-to-one ACRA interventions. The same therapist completes the work.

Session 1: Caregiver introduction and motivation

In this first session the therapist aims to increase parents' motivation to work on the problem by instilling hope. Parents are encouraged to follow the points given here.
- Consider stopping their own substance use, but certainly avoiding substance use and intoxication in the presence of adolescents, thus modelling the behaviour they desire. According to ACRA this is the single most important action for parents.

- Develop positive communication. Criticising, blame and negativity are unhelpful, even when messages being communicated are appropriate. Maintaining a solution-focused, strengths-based response is more effective. ACRA includes a 'daily reminder to be nice' for all involved.
- Parents are encouraged to actively monitor their child's whereabouts and whom they are with.
- Help the teen engage in healthy, non-drug-oriented, prosocial activities.

Session 2: Caregiver communication skills

Under stress we can respond in ways that increase rather than decrease tensions. ACRA communication techniques include:

- making an understanding statement (e.g. 'I know this party is important to you')
- taking partial responsibility (e.g. 'I'm sorry I sometimes lose my temper')
- offering to help (e.g. 'What about going out on Saturday night instead?').

If a teenager asks to go to a party, rather than simply saying 'no' a parent can say something like:

> Tom, I know you think I'm being hard on you and maybe I am being cautious. However, you got in trouble at school for smoking a joint so you can't go to a party. If things go okay for 2 weeks, you can go to the next one.

Session 3: Joint session to practise relationship skills

In the third appointment the adolescent and parent practise together the skills they have been learning separately. These include communication and problem-solving skills. During the session they discuss aspects of the relationship they are both happy with and aspects they would like to improve.

Non-Violent Resistance model

The NVR model supports parents to make changes in the family home where violence towards them by an adolescent is present. Violence is resisted peacefully. While this may not be a problem for every parent, many are silently managing violence in their home. This might be related to desire for drugs or alcohol, withdrawal effects or drug debts. The degree of violence is not important, as even the threat of violence can be sufficient to immobilise parents. The NVR model was inspired by peaceful protests carried out as a resistance to dominating actions and systems at a political level.[12–14] Parents begin this process by letting the young person know that violence will not be used or tolerated in the home.[13] NVR involves moving closer to the teen, physically and emotionally, rather than moving away from their oppositional behaviour. NVR proposes resistance techniques, including those outlined here.

- Making a formal announcement that unacceptable behaviours will be responded to by resistance.
- Parents develop a list of supporters who become involved in 'sit-ins' and are available to come to the home to join the peaceful protest.
- Carrying out 'sit-ins' to demonstrate their commitment to change.
- Violent behaviour will be documented and given to the adolescent after the incident so that they can read the impact of their actions.
- Creature comforts of the family home will be withdrawn, if violent or unacceptable behaviour persists.

Parents are encouraged to recognise where they are being drawn into patterns of argument that escalate. A goal of NVR is to identify ways to short circuit these patterns. NVR strategies include those outlined here.

- Delaying response to unacceptable behaviours. Omer and colleagues[13] recommend brief phrases that act as reminders, such as, 'Strike while the iron is cold', to help parents slow things down.
- 'You don't need to win, but only to persevere' is another phrase that reminds parents that they don't need to have the last word.
- Avoiding 'ping-pong' arguments helps parents avoid joining in an escalation.
- NVR sees self-control as strength and encourages parents to practise it.

CONCLUSION

Often parents have been working in a determined way to deal with adolescent drug misuse for some time before they contact any service. Parents may not seek help initially because of stigma, shame, hopelessness or the experience of feeling blamed. Practitioners who notice indicators that substance misuse may be causing problems can do much to support parents as they address their concerns. Taking time to identify and emphasise parents' own resources bolsters the family system. There is evidence that parental influence can reduce the risks of adolescents becoming involved in substance misuse. This important influence can also reduce or reverse the risk trajectory for teenagers who are misusing substances. Parents will probably be the most significant influence in a teen's decision to stop problematic drug or alcohol use.

KEY POINTS

- Adolescent substance misuse problems are positively affected by parental efforts to reduce them.
- Adolescents do not need to agree with their parents' standpoint to be positively influenced.
- Even if an adolescent does not want to change his or her substance misuse, parents can be the change agent.
- Support from friends, community and professionals can be helpful in dealing with these problems.

FURTHER READING

➡ National Treatment Agency for Substance Misuse; Building Recovery in Communities. *Substance Misuse among Young People 2011–12*. London: National Health Service; 2012. Available at: www.nta.nhs.uk/uploads/yp2012vfinal.pdf

➡ *Narrative therapy*: the Dulwich Centre provides a wealth of information on narrative therapy (www.dulwichcentre.com.au/).

➡ *ACRA*: the manual used in the Cannabis Youth Treatment study is available online at: www.dldocs.stir.ac.uk/documents/ACRA_CYT_v4.pdf. It provides a detailed breakdown of the sessions and techniques within this model.

REFERENCES

1 Home Office, UK. *Drug Strategy 2010: reducing demand, restricting supply, building recovery; supporting people to live a drug free life*. London: Home Office; 2010.

2 Velleman R, Bradbury C. *Supporting and Involving Carers: a guide for commissioners and providers*. London: National Treatment Agency for Substance Misuse; 2008. Available at: www.nta.nhs.uk/uploads/supporting_and_involving_carers2008_0509. pdf (accessed 10 August 2013).

3 Carr A. The effectiveness of family therapy and systemic interventions for child-focused problems. *J Fam Ther*. 2009; **31**(1): 3–45.

4 Hogue A, Liddle H A. Family-based treatment for adolescent substance abuse: controlled trials and new horizons in services research. *J Fam Ther*. 2009; **31**(2): 126–54.

5 Tanner-Smith EE, Wilson SJ, Lipsey MW. The comparative effectiveness of outpatient treatment for adolescent substance abuse: a meta-analysis. *J Subst Abuse Treat*. 2013; **44**(2): 145–58.

6 Olszewski D, Burkhart G, Bo A. *Children's Voices: experiences and perceptions of European children on drug and alcohol issues*. Luxembourg: The Publications Office of the European Union; 2010.

7 Usher K, Jackson D, O'Brien L. Shattered dreams: parental experiences of adolescent substance abuse. *Int J Ment Health Nurs*. 2007; **16**(6): 422–30.

8 Dallos R, Urry A. Abandoning our parents and grandparents: does social construction mean the end of systemic family therapy? *J Fam Ther.* 1999; **21**(2): 161–86.

9 Epston D, White M, Murray K. A proposal for a re-authoring therapy: Rose's revisioning of her life and a commentary. In: McNamee S, Gergen KJ, editors. *Therapy as Social Construction.* London: Sage; 1993. pp. 96–115.

10 White M. *Maps of Narrative Practice.* New York, NY: WW Norton; 2007.

11 Godley SH, Myers RJ, Smith JE, *et al. The Adolescent Community Reinforcement Approach for Adolescent Cannabis Users, Cannabis Youth Treatment (CYT) Series.* Volume 4. DHHS Pub. No. 01–3489. Rockville, MD: Center for Substance Abuse Treatment; Substance Abuse and Mental Health Services Administration; 2001.

12 Omer H. *Nonviolent Resistance: a new approach to violent and self-destructive children.* New York, NY: Cambridge University Press; 2004.

13 Omer H, Schorr-Sapir I, Weinblatt U. Non-violent resistance and violence against siblings. *J Fam Ther.* 2008; **30**(4): 450–64.

14 Lebowitz E, Dolberger D, Nortov E, *et al.* Parent training in nonviolent resistance for adult entitled dependence. *Fam Process.* 2012; **51**(1): 90–106.

CHAPTER 9

Enhancing motivation for change

INTRODUCTION

Change is difficult. It's hard for adults, let alone adolescents. It's rare to find teenagers who present with high motivation to change their substance use. When working with adolescents, professionals need to remember a simple fact: you cannot make a teenager change. If the adolescent is to change it will be because he or she becomes determined to change. Therefore, professionals working with youth need a good understanding of what *does* and *does not* work when it comes to enhancing motivation. In this chapter, an overview of Motivational Interviewing (MI) will be presented. MI is a well-researched, widely used strategy for motivating individuals in the area of goal-oriented change. Our aim is to equip professionals with a working understanding of the model and some basic information about the skills that will help motivate teenagers.

AN OVERVIEW OF MOTIVATIONAL INTERVIEWING

MI is one of the most widely used strategies to increase motivation. It has been adapted for use in a range of settings including medical, youth work, forensic services, public health and psychiatric services. MI is a client-centred, directive method for increasing motivation by exploring and resolving ambivalence.[1] It was developed in 1983 by William Miller for the treatment of problem drinking. It was further developed in collaboration with Dr Stephen Rollnick.

What is motivation?

Motivation can be described as the series of inner processes that guide, direct and keep us focused on goal-oriented behavioural change. At a fundamental level, it's the reason somebody has for using certain behaviours, or it could be seen as a general willingness to do something. Historically, motivation was viewed as a fixed personality characteristic.[2] From a clinical perspective, motivation was viewed as being the client's responsibility and not the professional's.[1] When clients were unmotivated, they were labelled as resistant. MI takes a different view. Instead, when resistance happens in the professional relationship, the worker sees that they need to do something different. In MI, motivation is viewed as being on a continuum. It isn't a fixed element, thus it can increase or decrease.

Why does increased motivation help teens?

There are many reasons why it helps to be motivated. Those who are motivated are more likely to work on their problems. The more motivated one is, the more time and effort they will put into the goals they set. Motivation is directly correlated with better outcomes. Apart from the direct benefit to individuals, motivation is linked to better outcomes for staff and governments. Motivated teenagers are easier and more enjoyable to work with, leading to less burnout among staff. Furthermore, they are less costly to services and state.[3]

Ambivalence and change

> I love the feeling of being stoned. I don't have to think about anything . . . but I am so fed up of getting arrested and fighting with my parents.
>
> —*John, aged 16*

Sometimes people don't want to change, but sometimes, they do *and* they don't want to. Ambivalence is the feeling of wanting two conflicting things. In relation to substance use, it is often described as the 'I want to stop but I don't want to stop' dilemma. It is a completely normal process.

In addition to a desire to stop, Miller and Rollnick[1] suggest that a person's confidence in his or her ability to stop plays an important role in motivation. They suggest four different possible profiles of clients who may attend.

In the 1980s, James Prochaska and Carlo DiClemente developed their transtheoretical model. They proposed a framework for conceptualising the change process. In this approach, change is seen as a fluctuating process, with different stages. At each stage, the worker has a specific set of tasks that will facilitate clients' movements through the process.

The do's and don't's of motivation

Historically, treatment providers were under the impression that they had to beat their clients into accepting they had a problem. Denial was the enemy. The good old-fashioned 'we'll break you down and then build you back up'

TABLE 9.1 Four client profiles[1]

Low Importance, High Confidence	Individuals who fit this profile believe they could change if they wanted to, but ultimately don't want to
Low Importance, Low Confidence	These clients don't view change as being important, but even if they did, they don't believe they could change
High Importance, Low Confidence	This group recognise that change is desirable and important, but their confidence is low; they don't believe they can make the changes they want to make
High Importance, High Confidence	Here is the ideal situation; an individual wants to change, they believe change is important and they have faith in their ability to make the changes they are seeking

approach was used in many services. Thankfully, we've moved on from that. Today, evidence-based approaches are the norm and service providers meet their clients with respect and understanding. MI is the most commonly used approach and seeks to elicit 'change talk' from the client. Through skilled reflective listening, and the application of a range of skills, we encourage clients to make statements about their reasons for changing. These statements are referred to as 'change talk' and the more change talk a client engages in the more motivated they become. For example, a teen saying, 'I only drink the same as my friends' is getting less motivated. However, a young person saying, 'I don't seem to handle drinking as well as my friends' is getting more motivated. The analogy of 'dancing not wrestling' is one way of conceptualising the work. When we think of wrestling, a battle immediately comes to mind. The two participants are fighting for dominance, whereas dancers work together, moving in accord to achieve their goal. According to Miller and Rollinick,[1] there are four principles to MI:

1 express empathy
2 develop discrepancy
3 roll with resistance
4 promote self-efficacy.

Empathy

Carl Rogers[5] defined empathy as trying to accurately perceive the world and experiences of others. There is much evidence to support its use in helping relationships. Feeling heard is central to the therapeutic process. When we are empathic, we are striving to understand the client from their point of view. By its nature, it is non-judgemental. We don't have to condone adolescents' behaviours, but neither should we criticise the choices they make.[6] Empathy is communicated through skilful reflective listening. Paraphrasing, summarising and reflection of feeling are all ways we can convey empathy.

TABLE 9.2 The Stages of Change[4]

Stage	Description	Task for professionals
Precontemplation	This is the earliest stage of change. Here the teen isn't even considering changing his or her behaviour. The teen may not realise he or she has a problem or doesn't see his or her behaviour as unhealthy. Pre-contemplators can be 'Reluctant, Resigned, Rebellious or Rationalise their behaviour.'[4]	As professionals, it's our job to listen carefully, provide feedback in an empathic manner and raise awareness about the possibility of risk. We strive to instil hope, respect the client's autonomy and explore obstacles to change.
Contemplation	Contemplation is the second stage. It is characterised by ambivalence. Here the adolescent knows he or she has a problem and is considering making a change. The person knows where he or she is and where he or she wants to be, but may still balk at making the commitment to change.	In this stage, our task is to examine the length of time the adolescent has been thinking about change, provide information and feedback. We facilitate an exploration of the risks of drug use and the benefits of changing. Essentially, we examine the pros and cons and seek to tip the balance in the favour of change without coercion.
Preparation	Here the client accepts change is necessary. He or she is described as being 'on the verge of taking action.'[4] The client will either take the step into action or go back into the contemplation stage.	Here our role is to help the client to figure out the best course of action. Work on a plan that is specific, measured, acceptable, accessible, timed, appropriate, doable and effective.
Action	In this stage, the person is doing something to make change happen. Essentially, the person puts their plan into action. This phase requires effort, determination and takes time and energy.	Clients need support in taking necessary steps. Affirmation, listening skills, exploration of options and additional supports may be required. We strive to build the client's self-efficacy.
Maintenance and Relapse	Maintenance is viewed as the final step in the change process. The young person works to build on successes and too often battles with relapse. The transtheoretical model views it as a continuum that can last a lifetime. Relapse is possible (likely) and recommitment is often needed.	Our work here consists of helping the client to develop relapse prevention skills and help them revisit the process of contemplation, preparation and action if relapse occurs. Encouragement is vital.

Gerald Egan[7] suggests a basic formula for conveying empathy: 'You feel . . . because . . .'

Teenager: It's really hard. My friends don't understand. They say I'm boring when I'm not drinking. I go out and it's like I'm on a different wave length. I'm there, but I'm not there. They're all pissed enjoying themselves and I'm sitting there watching them but it's like I'm alone.

Worker: Sounds like *you're feeling* lonely *because* you're not operating on the same level as they are while they're drunk. It's like you're not connecting with them at the time. And you're really struggling with it at the moment.

Develop discrepancy

Discrepancies are gaps between clients' current behaviour and goals they have. Essentially, it's the difference between where the adolescent is and where he or she wants to be. Adolescents who have a strong desire to finish school might experience feelings of unease when they realise that their cannabis use is having a negative impact on their ability to concentrate. These uncomfortable feelings can motivate the teenager to make changes. In MI, the professional reflects these discrepancies to the young person.

Remember, we are listening for the client's arguments for change. It can be tempting to point out all the arguments for change we observe, but skilful reflection of *the client's* change talk is more powerful. One useful tool is the cost-benefit analysis. Asking clients to complete one can help them, and you, to reflect on the reasons for and against change. You will find free and accessible cost-benefit worksheets available on many websites.

TABLE 9.3 Example of a cost-benefit analysis

The good things about my cannabis use are:	The not-so-good things about my cannabis use are:
The good things about changing my cannabis use are:	The not-so-good things about changing my cannabis use are:

Roll with resistance

In previous approaches to substance misuse treatment, when individuals presented arguments against change, workers built up a healthy sweat trying to argue for it. All that achieves is red-faced professionals and frustrated clients. In MI, we are encouraged to roll with resistance. The stronger we argue for change, the stronger they argue against it. Techniques to deal with resistance will be presented later. For now, remember the following five principles[1]:

1 avoid arguing for change
2 don't directly oppose resistance
3 invite new perspectives, but don't impose them
4 look to the teenager for solutions
5 if resistance is present, use it as a signal to try something different.

Support self-efficacy

Self-efficacy is the person's confidence in his or her ability to complete a specific task. It is different from general confidence. For example, a confident person who can easily present workshops may have no belief in his or her ability to stop smoking. Research tells us self-efficacy is a good predictor of change, therefore it's vital in motivation. If an adolescent believes he or she can change, it will have a direct impact on the effort the adolescent makes to change. Using a confidence ruler is one way of assessing how confident a client is about a proposed change.

No confidence									Completely confident
1	2	3	4	5	6	7	8	9	10

The higher they rate themselves on the ruler, the more likely they are to make the change, assuming the change is one they wish to make. A low confidence rating suggests we need to focus on building self-efficacy. Sending clients out with a plan they're not confident they can achieve (no matter how badly they want it) is setting them up to fail. Self-efficacy is built when the client sets realistic goals and achieves them. More challenging goals can follow gradually. Kadden and Sample[8] suggest exploring the past for previous successes and accomplishments as a way of increasing self-efficacy.

BOX 9.1 Key points

1 Work on empathising – try to understand the teenager and communicate this understanding.
2 Develop discrepancy – use the information you are hearing to reflect any differences between the teen's goals and his or her current behaviour.
3 Avoid arguing! Avoid arguing! Avoid arguing! It doesn't work.
4 Support self-efficacy – work with the young person to build their confidence in his or her ability to make the chances he or she wants to make.

Skills used in motivational interviewing

One of the most important elements of MI is the elicitation of change talk. Change talk consists of statements clients make that are in essence, arguments for change. Miller and Rollnick[1] describe it as 'self-motivating speech'. The mnemonic DARN-C is suggested as a way to remember what we are listening out for.[9]

D = Desire statements: 'I want to stop taking coke.'

A = Ability statements: 'If I wanted to stop, I could.'

R = Reason statements: 'I'm going to fail my exams if I don't get it together.'

N = Need statements: 'I need to give clean urines for the judge.'

C = Commitment statements: 'I'm going to give this a real go.'

Whenever you hear change talk, reflect it back to the young person. The goal is to let them hear the arguments *he or she* is making for change.

Traps to avoid

Before we explore the necessary skills of MI, let's take a look at what doesn't help. There are certain traps professionals working with substance use fall in to. If we remember that our primary goal is to elicit change talk, there are certain techniques that don't work. The main mistakes therapists make regarding attempts to motivate clients are as follows.[1]

The question–answer trap

Nobody wants to be interrogated. If we fire question after question, then we run the risk of trying to control the session, alienating the client and ultimately, destroying the opportunity for motivation. There are times when we fall into this trap. Let's see what it might look like.

Worker: So you've been smoking a bit of weed?

Client: Yeah.

Worker: And your parents are a bit worried about this?

Client: I guess.

Worker: Are you worried about it?

Client: No.

Worker: Do you smoke every day?

Client: Pretty much.

Not the most stimulating conversation in the world, right? Not only is the worker failing to connect with the client, they are basically only eliciting one-word answers, and no change talk is presented. Firing question after question at teenagers doesn't work, especially closed questions. If you need specific information, then a closed question might be appropriate, but a good rule of thumb is to avoid asking them. This chapter offers you other skills to use that can be interspersed with questions so that you can avoid the trap of interrogating clients.

Taking sides

In Miller and Rollnick's[1] book, this is the trap that we are told is the most important to avoid. In its usual form, this trap presents itself when the worker hears the adolescent making some statement that indicates the presence of a problem and tells the young person why it's a problem and what they need to do about it. Here's what it looks like.

Worker: Wow, you've been arrested twice for being drunk and disorderly this month? That's not good. Maybe you need to seriously rethink your drinking.

Client: I had three cans and was singing on the street. It's not like I was beating someone up. The police overreact about these things. I'm not a total dipso.

Remember, *if we argue for change, the client will argue against it!* If you remember that change talk should come from the client, you might avoid this trap. Furthermore, research actually shows that the more arguments for change professionals make, the less likely change is to occur.

The labelling trap

We are there to support, guide, encourage and facilitate. Not to label. Avoiding labels is advisable with any client in substance misuse discussions, but it's especially important with adolescents. Labelling runs the risk of leading to the taking sides trap. Unless the client wants to embrace a label, then stay away from it. Telling adolescents they are addicts or alcoholics is one strategy that is likely to evoke arguments against change from the client. Problems can be explored without labelling them.

The expert trap

We are not there to fix clients, and ultimately, they know far more about their life hopes and struggles than we do. If we adopt the position of expert, the client is likely to fall into a passive role. We don't want this. We want them engaged in the process. Remember, the spirit of MI suggests collaboration. An expert position doesn't promote this.

The premature focus trap

As professionals, we have a desire to help clients. However, clients will have their own thoughts on what they want to address. One trap we fall into is trying to put the focus on what we see as the problem. Miller and Rollnick[1] remind us that sometimes talking about the concerns that are pressing to the client will bring us back to the topic that concerns us as workers. Don't focus too early on the 'problem' of substance use. Instead, listen and explore current concerns and this will generally lead back to the substance use without alienating the client.

Blaming trap

Another trap that poses the possibility of ensnaring us is blaming. It's not important whose *fault* the 'problem' is. It's likely that many significant people in the adolescent's life are already blaming their substance use for everything. In MI, we operate a 'no-fault' policy. We aren't looking to blame anyone for the problem. Instead, we're there to support the young person to make the changes they want to make.

Skills to practise

So now that we've considered what not to do, let's explore some of the skills that help to evoke change talk. OARS is a commonly used mnemonic to help workers remember the core skills necessary in Motivational Interviewing.[1]

O = Open questions
A = Affirmation
R = Reflection
S = Summarising

Open questions

Open-ended questions are designed to elicit the maximum answer. They are questions that are difficult to answer in a monosyllabic manner. Who? What? Where? and When? are examples of questions that are more likely to get the client talking. Statements such as 'tell me about', or 'describe for me' are also useful prefaces to questions. The use of 'do you', 'would you' and 'is/are' tend to start closed ended questions. Open questions can be used at every stage of the process. The aim is to elicit change talk. This is where MI is more directive. We can choose carefully the questions that are likely to elicit arguments for change. Ask an open question and try to follow it up with reflective listening or minimal encouragers (hmmm, nodding, uh-huh, and so forth) rather than firing another question at the adolescent.

Closed question	Open question
Worker: Do you smoke cannabis?	Worker: Tell me about your cannabis use?
Client: Yes	Client: Well, I started when I was twelve. I tend to smoke it mostly when I'm with my friends but lately, I've noticed I'm using it on my own in my bedroom.

Food for thought

Think about the questions you usually use with clients. Are they open or closed? How can you obtain the information you need to get, without falling into the question–answer trap? Actively work on ways to open up questions. Elicit maximum information with minimal intervention. It's a skill. *Practise it.*

Affirmation

As previously stated, change is difficult. A little affirmation goes a long way. However, we never want to appear condescending, so by affirmation we're not talking about 'Pollyanna-ish' patronising statements that don't ring true. Instead, use reflection to acknowledge progress, appreciate how difficult things can be and affirm strengths the client has.

Reflective listening

This is one of the most important things we can do, especially with adolescents. Everyone wants to be heard and understood. Reflective listening allows us to convey that we are listening and trying to grasp and understand their experiences, feelings or behaviours. A key skill is to be tentative in your reflections. Don't assume you understand; instead, check it out with the young person. Useful openers to reflective listening include:
'It sounds like . . .'
'Am I hearing you say . . .'
'It seems as though you're saying . . .'

The use of a questioning tone at the end of a statement is another way of being tentative. Make the reflection in statement form, but raise your tone, so that the adolescent knows it's a question, not a blanket assumption that you've picked them up correctly. Alternatively, reflect back what you think your client is communicating and then ask, 'Have I got that right?'

When considering reflection, avoid parroting. Nobody wants to hear their words back over and over again. Develop the skill of paraphrasing. Think about your client's statements and offer them back in your own words. Another thing to bear in mind is *what* you reflect back. Anytime you hear change talk (remember DARN-C) you reflect it. This allows clients to re-hear their own arguments for change.

The best way to become proficient at these skills is to practise them, as much and as often as you can.

Practice Exercise 9.1

Think about ways you could reflect the following statements:

'Sometimes I wish I could drink like everyone else. You know, go out and have a few bottles and not pick up new charges.'

'I'd like to stop. I think it would be really hard, but I'd like to. At least then my parents would be off my back.'

'I am sick of my probation officer being on my case. Every time I see her she has something to say.'

Summarising

Summaries should be used consistently. They do a number of things. Firstly, as a professional having a conversation with a young person, we will gather a lot of important information. Summarising periodically helps us stay on track and ensure we don't miss key information. Secondly, we are reflecting change talk to the individual. We do it routinely as we paraphrase and listen reflectively. Summaries provide us with opportunity to reinforce arguments the person makes for change. There are three types of summaries suggested in MI.

1 Collection summaries

These summaries are used when we are exploring with the teenager. Miller and Rollnick[10] use the analogy of flowers to describe collection summaries. Each time the young person makes a change talk statement, it's like one flower being collected by the professional. After we hear a few, we offer the young person a bouquet of change talk, letting them hear his or her own desire, ability, reason, need and commitment statements. These summaries are short and are designed to convey we are listening and understanding, but are also used to gather more information. It's common to hear the brief collecting summary followed by a gentle probe such as 'what else?' or 'tell me more about that.'

2 Linking summaries

Linking summaries are useful when we bring together different pieces of the teenager's story. Think of it as weaving separate threads into one cohesive braid. The purpose of linking summaries is to encourage the young person to reflect on the common aspects of two or more pieces of information. A good example of a linking summary is when we reflect ambivalence. We offer back the reasons for and against change that the teen has presented. We are essentially summarising the positives and negatives the young person has discussed with us. Linking summaries can also be useful when we are making links in relation to patterns. Perhaps we hear the teen tell us about a drinking episode that ended in a fight and we are reminded of a similar story he or she told us. Phrases such as 'On one hand . . . and on the other . . .' can be useful.

3 Transitional summaries

The third type of summary used in MI is the transitional summary. This does exactly what it says on the tin. It's used when you are transitioning from one stage of the process to the next. You are bringing together everything that has been discussed in one final summary before you move on to the next piece of the picture. They are useful at the end of an assessment process, or indeed the end of a session, but can also be used when there is a logical movement from one aspect of the young person's story to the next within an individual session.

Evoking change talk

While the OARS will help you begin the exploration of change talk with a teenager, MI also suggests specific interventions that can be used to elicit arguments for change.

Asking evocative questions

Ultimately, with this approach to motivation we are eliciting change talk. Asking directly is easiest. Remember your DARN-C when formulating evocative questions. Miller and Rollnick[1] suggest asking open-ended questions that explore the following:

- Disadvantages of the status quo (reason statements)
  — *What are the not-so-good things about your heroin use?*
- Advantages of change (need statements)
  — *What would be different if you weren't using heroin?*
- Optimism about change (ability statements)
  — *What changes have you already made and what helped with this?*
- Intention to change (commitment statements)
  — *So what could you do differently in this case?*

Practice Exercise 9.2

Brainstorm a list of questions you can use when you're working with young people. Look for open-ended questions that are likely to elicit a change talk response.

Other strategies suggested in MI include using rulers. Earlier in this chapter, a confidence ruler was demonstrated to explore a teenager's self-efficacy. This ruler can also be used to initiate conversation about the importance of change. Miller and Rollnick[1] offer two questions that can be used in conjunction with the ruler:

1 'Why are you a _____ and not at zero?'
2 'What would have to be different for you to go from ____ to a higher number?'

The cost-benefit analysis is another way we can explore the pros and cons of an adolescent's substance use. Remember, he or she will have very good reasons for using and for not using.

Resistance in the Motivational Interviewing process

MI takes a different stance to other therapeutic styles with regard to resistance in the helping relationship. Instead of labelling clients 'resistant', professionals view resistance as a sign they need to change tack. Miller and Rollnick[10] joke that historically, therapists have proposed that when the client disagrees with them, it's viewed as resistance and when the client agrees with the professional, it is insight. Remember when we encounter resistance in our helping relationships, it's a definite signal that things aren't going well. If resistance is present, then collaboration is absent, and MI believes that collaboration is vital. When you get that sense of argument, pause, reflect on what you're doing and try a different strategy.

Working with resistance

In their professional training video, Miller and Rollnick[10] offer a list of signs that tell us resistance is occurring in the therapeutic relationship. First and foremost, we are told that resistance looks like arguing. There will be a sense of disagreement or discord between worker and client, with the worker usually trying to coerce the client into seeing things their way.

Other forms of resistance include tuning out, interruption, ignoring, coming late or missing sessions, passivity or overt behaviours that the client uses to let us know they're not happy. Trust us, you'll know when resistance is there. So what do you do about it? Bearing in mind that it's our responsibility to adapt

when resistance is present, MI offers strategies and techniques we can use to 'roll with resistance'. In this approach, we can respond reflectively or strategically. So let's start with reflective responses. According to Miller and Rollinick[10] there are three types of reflections we can use when we meet resistance:
1 simple reflection
2 amplified reflection
3 double-sided reflection.

Simple reflection

Here the worker simply paraphrases or reflects what the client has said. The aim is to convey a sense of understanding. Empathy is powerful in the face of resistance, especially if the teenager is expecting an argument.

Client: This is stupid. I don't need to be here. I don't have a problem. I swear, my parents are stuck in the Stone Age. It was just one joint. I don't need counselling.

Worker: So from where you're sitting, you feel your parents overreacted to your use of cannabis. You really don't see a value in being here.

Amplified reflection

With amplified reflections, the worker again reflects what they hear the young person saying, but they amplify the reflection. Essentially, we reflect what the person is arguing but amp up the intensity of it. In fact, we are amplifying the very thing we might want to oppose. Something strange happens when we do this. The adolescent sometimes backtracks and changes their stance on the original statement they made.

Client: Seriously, it's a bit of weed. It's not like heroin. It's not going to kill me. I don't see anything wrong with it. It calms me down.

Worker: So in your eyes, cannabis is completely safe and doesn't have any harmful consequences. In fact, you see it as being good for you.

Client: Well, I probably wouldn't say 'good for me.' It does make me paranoid.

Double-sided reflection

Double-sided reflections are important interventions for reflecting ambivalence. If a person's recent statement only presents the resistant side of an argument, a double-sided reflection takes what the client has said and adds to it the other side of the ambivalence. This is where linking summaries become useful. You may have to use information the client has previously given you to reflect both sides of the ambivalence.[10]

Strategic ways of responding to resistance

Shifting focus

This is the most obvious way to deal with resistance. We simply change the focus. Why waste time battling to get the adolescent talking about something they obviously don't want to talk about?

Client: I don't want to be here. I can't believe the judge said I had to get counselling. I just take coke the odd time. It's not a big deal.

Worker: I'm hearing you say your drug use isn't an issue for you. If you do have to come for the next 6 weeks, what would you like to talk about?

Reframing

Reframing is another way to deal with resistance. Here, the professional attempts to change the meaning of what the adolescent is sharing. It allows the teenager to see things differently.

Client: It's not that I haven't tried before. I have. I've tried over and over again. It's just so hard. All my friends drink. It's impossible to go out with them and not have a few bottles.

Worker: What strikes me is how persistent you are. You keep trying. That suggests this change is important to you. You haven't given up.

Emphasising personal choice

When people feel their freedom is being threatened, independence becomes more important. This is especially true in adolescents where one of the developmental tasks is that struggle for autonomy. The best thing to do is to emphasise that you, or anyone else for that matter, can't make them change, and so you won't try. In the end, it is the adolescent who determines what happens. The client's decisions are paramount. There's no point in fighting it. All we can do is assure them that they do in fact have the power of choice.

Siding with the negative

This is a strategy we use whereby we side with the negative, thus allowing the client to argue for change. It's one we have to be careful with. Use it only when you've established a good working relationship with your client. This ensures you don't run the risk of coming across as sarcastic.

No matter how we choose to respond to resistance, MI encourages us to move alongside the client. Ultimately, we want the process to be effective, and argument never is!

CONCLUSION

Miller and Rollinick's book *Motivational Interviewing* is a sound investment for any professional working with adolescents. Motivational Interviewing is one of the best methods we can employ to help motivate clients. It is a simple, yet powerful way of working with teenagers. Remember, that many adolescents will already have plenty of 'well meaning' adults telling them why they should change. Be someone different; be the person who strives to help them come to their own realisations of why change may be beneficial.

KEY POINTS

- MI is a way of working with people that promotes personal responsibility and increases motivation.
- As professionals, we strive to elicit change talk from clients.
- Whenever you hear change talk, reflect, reflect, reflect!
- Never ever, argue for change. It is a losing battle that can do real harm.
- Empathise with the teenager. Seek to get a real understanding of how they feel and how they see their own behaviour.
- Use open questions, affirmation, reflective responses and summarising to build the relationship with the teenager, and to help resolve their ambivalence.
- Work on ways of developing discrepancy. Help the client evaluate if what they are doing is getting them what they want.
- Remember self-efficacy. Sometimes helping a client increase their confidence in their ability to change is the primary task.
- When resistance is present in the relationship, adopt a different approach.

FURTHER READING

➡ Naar-King S, Suarez M. *Motivational Interviewing with Adolescents and Young Adults: applications of Motivational Interviewing.* New York, NY: Guilford Press; 2010.

REFERENCES

1 Miller WR, Rollnick S. *Motivational Interviewing: preparing people to change addictive behavior.* 2nd ed. New York, NY: Guilford Press; 2002.
2 Walters ST, Clark MD, Gingerich R, *et al. Motivating Offenders to Change: a guide for probation and parole.* CreateSpace Independent Publishing Platform; 2007.
3 Hayes TL, Ruthig JC, Perry RP, *et al.* Reducing the academic risks of over-optimism: the longitudinal effects of attributional retraining on cognition and achievement. *Res High Educ.* 2006; 47(7): 755–79.

4 DiClemente CC, Marden-Velasquez M. Motivational Interviewing and the stages of change. In: Miller WR, Rollnick S, editors. *Motivational Interviewing: preparing people to change addictive behaviour.* New York, NY: Guilford Press; 1991. pp. 191–202.

5 Rogers C. Empathic: an unappreciated way of being. *Couns Psychol.* 1975; 5(2): 2–10.

6 Arkowitz H, Westra HA, Miller WR, *et al. Motivational Interviewing in the Treatment of Psychological Problems.* New York, NY: Guilford Press; 2007.

7 Egan G. *The Skilled Helper: a systematic approach to effective helping.* 3rd ed. Monterey, CA: Thomson Brooks/Cole; 1986.

8 Sampl S, Kadden R. *Motivational Enhancement Therapy and Cognitive Behavioural Therapy for Adolescent Cannabis Users: 5 sessions.* Rockville, MD: US Department of Health and Human Services; 2001.

9 Sciacca K. *Motivational Interviewing: MI, glossary and fact sheet.* New York, NY: Sciacca Comprehensive Service Development for Mental Illness, Drug Addiction and Alcoholism; 2009. Available at: www.motivationalinterview.net/miglossary.pdf (accessed 11 August 2013).

10 Miller WR, Rollnick S. *Motivational Interviewing Professional Training* [DVD]. Albuquerque: University of New Mexico; 1998.

CHAPTER 10

Counselling adolescent substance users

INTRODUCTION

While counselling is a profession in and of itself, some of the skills used by therapists are applicable to anyone working with adolescents. In counselling, connection and relationship building is important. This is particularly true for adolescents, and the ability to listen, empathise and engage in dialogue is vital for professionals working with adolescent substance users. In this chapter, readers will be introduced to the Adolescent Community Reinforcement Approach (ACRA). This is an evidence-based counselling style, designed specifically for work with adolescent substance users.

THEORETICAL BACKGROUND

Dr Robert J Meyers, an American psychologist, developed ACRA. It emerged from the Community Reinforcement Approach model, founded by George Hunt and Nathan Azran. In essence, it is a form of cognitive behavioural therapy. With ACRA, substance misuse is viewed as a learned behaviour. In this section, readers will be presented with a brief overview of the theoretical concepts and how they relate to substance use. The ACRA approach and some of the inherent procedures are then presented.

Cues and triggers for drug use

Much of the literature regarding substance use suggests craving is strongly associated with cues.[1-4] It is important to note that cues for use are unique to every client and thus cue identification will be a major part of any treatment approach influenced by the behaviour model.

With ACRA, the worker will understand that a young person's substance use behaviour doesn't exist in a vacuum. Instead, a range of antecedent cues commonly referred to as 'triggers' exist. Take, for example, the young person who repeatedly smokes cannabis to a soundtrack of reggae music. After a while, as soon as the adolescent hears the music, he thinks about cannabis use, which triggers a craving. Likewise, if an adolescent repeatedly pairs a mirror and bankcard with cocaine, eventually, simply seeing a mirror or card can engender the desire to use.

These triggers can consist of a range of external factors such as people, places, times, days, situations and a myriad of using paraphernalia. Likewise, triggers can be internal. Painful feelings such as grief, anxiety and anger can act as cues for drug use. If a teenager adopts a pattern of using whenever they experience difficult emotions, over time, those emotions become triggers. Internal cues are obviously more difficult to deal with. An adolescent can avoid certain people, places or things, but avoiding feelings is not as easy.

Operant conditioning

According to Heather and Robertson,[1] operant conditioning refers to the way in which the consequences of behaviour influence the likelihood of that behaviour being repeated. They inform us that there are four possible consequences to any behaviour.

1 *Positive reinforcement*: this refers to the positive outcome of the behaviour. The good feeling that someone gets from drinking alcohol reinforces the likelihood of drinking again.
2 *Negative reinforcement*: this refers to the manner in which the outcome of the behaviour increases the likelihood of repetition through avoidance of painful consequences. For example, a heroin user avoids the pain of withdrawal by using heroin, thus, the behaviour is reinforced.
3 *Punishment*: punishment relates to the painful consequences that occur through the use of a behaviour. For example, the cannabis smoker who repeatedly gets chest infections. In theory, the presence of these adverse consequences should reduce the likelihood of the behaviour being repeated.
4 *Response cost*: describes what happens when the expected outcome fails to occur. For example, if someone takes a dud acid tab and doesn't get high.

According to behaviour theories, the first two consequences are likely to increase the likelihood of the behaviour they follow. However, punishment and response cost are supposed to decrease the likelihood of the behaviour being repeated. When considering the negative consequences associated with substance use, it should make sense that the behaviour is discontinued following a health scare, legal difficulties, loss of relationships or other consequences of addiction. In reality, this is not the case. The reason for this is the immediacy of the reinforcements, as 'the punishing consequences come far too late.'[1] The immediate hit following ingestion of a drug outweighs the negative consequences that follow later.

THE ADOLESCENT COMMUNITY REINFORCEMENT APPROACH

ACRA draws on operant conditioning theories. Professionals utilise a set of procedures to identify the cues and triggers the adolescent has paired with substance use, as well as exploring the role of consequences in the drug use. Operant conditioning principles are also used in ACRA to actively identify what might be some reinforcers for prosocial behaviour.

In their 2001 manual, Goldley, *et al.*[5] identify the following goals of ACRA:

- the promotion of abstinence from cannabis, alcohol and other drugs
- the promotion of positive social activities
- healthy peer relationships
- better relationship within family.

As ACRA also includes some sessions with caregivers, goals of family sessions are as follows:

- helping caregivers to motivate the adolescent in the treatment process
- highlighting the role caregivers have in promoting abstinence
- providing caregivers with information relating to effective parenting.

Procedures

For trained ACRA therapists, this approach involves following a set of procedures designed to increase awareness, improve coping skills and encourage behaviour change. In its entirety, ACRA[6] comprises the following procedures:

- overview of ACRA
- functional analysis of substance-using behaviour
- functional analysis of prosocial (non-using behaviour)
- the Happiness Scale
- treatment plan/goals of counselling
- increasing prosocial recreation
- drink and drug refusal skills
- communication skills training (adolescent and caregiver versions)
- relapse prevention
- sobriety sampling
- problem-solving skills training (adolescent and caregiver versions)
- job-seeking skills
- anger management
- adolescent–caregiver relationship skills.

In a chapter this size, it would be impossible to explore each and every intervention used; however, a full explanation of the proceeding procedures can be found in the Cannabis Youth Treatment Series manual, *The Adolescent Community Reinforcement Approach for Adolescent Cannabis Users.*[5] This is a freely available manual with a lot of useful information about this evidence-based approach. Some of Meyers' publications are also presented in the references section at the end of this chapter.

Exploring some of the Adolescent Community Reinforcement Approach procedures

Assessment is the cornerstone of any treatment. In ACRA, the functional analysis (FA) is a vital component of assessment.

Functional analysis

An FA does exactly what it says on the tin. It analyses the function of a behaviour. In ACRA, there are two types of FAs completed with clients. The first is FA of their drug use behaviour, and the second follows later with a FA of a healthy, prosocial behaviour. The first FA is essentially a structured interview that explores the triggers and consequences of the substance use. It helps both the adolescent and the professional to identify the triggers leading up to the episode of use. Often, we hear clients tell us their drug use 'just happened'. However, in reality, there was probably a chain of events leading up to it – a chain consisting of many antecedent triggers. Second, it allows us to examine the positive and negative consequences of the behaviour. Remember, every behaviour is purposeful. There will be plenty of positive consequences. If adolescents didn't get something from using, they wouldn't keep doing it.

According to the Cannabis Youth Treatment Series manual,[5] 'the information gleaned from this process is never used in a confrontational manner.' Instead, our job is to help the young person put the consequences of their drug use into words. Godley, *et al.*[5] outline the following goals for the functional analysis:

- to help uncover reasons for changing the behaviour
- to highlight the fact that motivational factors for change are present
- to identify the triggers and their associated high-risk situations
- to clarify and bring greater awareness to the substance using behaviour
- to identify the short-term positive consequences to using
- to identify the long-term negative consequences to their drug use.

With adolescents, rapport-building is essential, so it's important to balance task and process. Eliciting the client's understanding as you explain the purpose can be a helpful way of involving them. We are encouraged to set positive expectations for treatment by telling the adolescent that ACRA is effective. Positive reinforcement is utilised throughout. Look for opportunities to affirm the teenager as you progress with the intervention. Even the smallest glimmer of motivation or attempts at change should be praised and reflected back to the young person.

On a practical level, the worker starts the process by explaining the purpose of the exercise:

> It would be helpful for us if I had a better understanding of your drug use and I'd like you to help me understand it. One way we can do this is to fill out a form called a *functional analysis*. Usually, people can pick out various things that lead up to drug use. We call them triggers. Triggers can be things outside of you, like mirrors and bankcards, or lighters, but they can also be things inside of you, like feelings, thoughts and memories. Once we've spent time exploring your triggers, we can then look at the positive and negative consequences of your drug use. So to start, will you describe a typical time when you used . . . (based on Godley, *et al.*[5])

Once you have buy-in from the adolescent, you explore his or her drug use with the FA form. Both client and professional have a copy in front of them for the duration of the session. Remember, the purpose of this intervention is fundamentally to define the problem behaviour.

BOX 10.1 Defining the behaviour using the functional analysis form

- List the times of day use occurs
- Identify the substances used
- Be specific about strengths of substances
- Be specific about amounts
- Explore circumstances in which the behaviour occurs
- Explore thoughts and feelings preceding the behaviour
- Identify relationships between people, places, things and times use occurs
- Explore the consequences (thoughts, feelings and actions following use) of the behaviour (both positive and negative)

Bearing this in mind, the worker uses open-ended questions to gather information about the internal and external triggers and the positive and negative consequences. It is suggested that we use the FA form as a guide. The last thing we want is to create an environment that feels like an interrogation. At every step of the ACRA process, bear in mind the importance of maintaining

Sample functional analysis form

External triggers	Internal triggers	Using behaviour	Positive consequences	Negative consequences

a connection. Box 10.2 presents a list of questions that you could use to assist in this process.

BOX 10.2 Questions to use in functional analyses

- Tell me about a typical day using
- What time do you first use?
- What exactly do you use?
- How much of it do you use?
- How do you use it?
- Where do you use it?
- How much do you spend on it?
- What goes through your head just before you use?
- What are some of the pleasant thoughts you have while using?
- How are you feeling before you use?
- What do you do just before you use?
- Who do you use with?
- Are there any times or situations where you are more likely to use?
- What happens after you use?
- What goes through your head after you use?
- How do you feel after you use?
- What do you do after you use?
- What's good about using?
- What's the not-so-good side of using?

With regard to the questions in Box 10.2, it can be really helpful to follow up the original question with further questions. Ensure you have the whole picture and use reflections to communicate you are trying to understand. It's a good idea to prepare a form that you can use with young people when completing this exercise. We've included a sample here that is based on the work of Meyers and Smith.[7] There are many pre-prepared worksheets available on the Internet, and a simple Google search will provide a variety to choose from.

The information the FA gathers is useful in a number of ways. Ultimately, strategies can be devised to influence the occurrence of the behaviour, either by decreasing it (in the case of problem behaviour) or increasing it (in the case of a healthy behaviour).[7] At the end of the intervention, we are armed with the following knowledge.

Client's triggers	This is helpful as it allows us to develop strategies that will help clients to either avoid, or learn to cope with exposure to the cues that have been identified.
Short-term positive consequences	Once we have this information, we can use it to help the client come up with alternative strategies for getting what they need. For example, if Johnny identified 'stress relief' as a short-term positive consequence of his weed use, we can build stress management into his coping plan and help him to learn healthier ways to get stress relief.
Long-term negative consequences	These give us motivational tools to use with clients. As we saw in the chapter on MI, reasons for change often involve the negative consequences of behaviour. Gaining greater insight into what a client sees as the downside of his or her using behaviour allows us to reflect back the client's own stated reasons for change.

It is important to summarise and paraphrase routinely as you complete the FA, and to ask some gentle probing questions to ensure you are getting the necessary information. ACRA suggests that we complete this procedure in the first and second session with the young person. However, it is a work in progress and will be revisited as the client makes changes in his or her life.[5]

BOX 10.3 Key point: functional analysis of substance use checklist[6]

- Explain the rationale for functional analysis
- Ask for a typical episode of use and explore in detail
- Explore internal and external cues
- Clarify the using behaviour
- Explore positive short-term consequences
- Explore negative long-term consequences
- Summarise the information gathered and outline how it will be used

Treatment planning

If the FA is used as an assessment process in ACRA, treatment planning comprises two intrinsically intertwined procedures: the Happiness Scale and the Goals of Counselling. The main aim of this procedure is to ascertain what the young person actually wants and help him or her plan to get it.

The Happiness Scale

The Happiness Scale comprises 16 areas of life that the adolescent is asked to consider on a scale of one to ten, with ten being completely happy and one being completely unhappy. Done early in the treatment process, it provides us with a baseline indication of the areas in which the young person may want to focus. While ACRA draws its theoretical underpinnings from a cognitive behavioural approach, here is where it is client centred in its delivery. It gives the young person the ability to reflect on and decide which areas of their life need to be addressed. The professional needs to explain the rationale for this intervention and give the adolescent clear, concise instructions regarding how they complete it. *See* Box 10.4 for Meyers'[6] suggestions for introducing the Happiness Scale.

BOX 10.4 Introducing the Happiness Scale

1   Explain the reason behind the scale:
   — outline that it helps the clients see what areas of their lives they're happy/ unhappy with
   — inform them that it highlight the aspects they want to work on in the counselling process, thus giving them choice and control in the process
   — explain how it gives an indication of change over time.
2   Give the client clear instructions as to how to complete the scale.
3   Review some of the circled ratings.

As far as self-reporting forms go, this one is easy to administer and adopts a holistic approach. Instead of focusing solely on substance use, the scale allows exploration of all areas of the client's life. However, it can of course be used to 'gently suggest, where appropriate, there could be a link between his or her using behaviour and unhappiness'.[5]

Rather than jumping straight into the areas the adolescent has indicated they're unhappy with, the worker first explores areas of strength. What has the adolescent circled as an area they're happy with? Focusing on what's going well builds rapport. It also highlights what strengths and resources the adolescent has. Once this is done, we focus on lower rated areas. It is suggested that we use the ratings as a vehicle to explore, in further detail, why the adolescent has rated things that way.[5] It might also be helpful to tease out why a client selected a 3 and not a 2. The fact that a client didn't score a 1 or a 2 suggests the situation has a lot of room for improvement, but it isn't completely negative either.

While the Happiness Scale is used in the first few sessions of the treatment process, it isn't a singular piece of work. ACRA suggests revisiting it every two weeks. This gives both client and professional insight into what external and internal factors might influence the shifts in scores on an ongoing basis. Clearly, the goal is progress. Change isn't a one-off event. There are small steps in the process and each should be explored and affirmed. Remember the R in ACRA stands for reinforcement, so use any and every opportunity that presents itself to reinforce change.

Sample Happiness Scale

Name: _____ Adolescent ID: _____ Date: _____

This scale is meant to estimate your current happiness with your life in each of the areas listed below. Please circle one of the numbers (1–10) beside each area. Numbers towards the left side indicate various degrees of unhappiness, whereas numbers towards the right side of the scale reflect increasing levels of happiness. Ask yourself this question as you rate each area of life: *'How happy am I today with this area of my life?'* In other words, state accordingly to the numerical scale (1–10) exactly how you feel today. Try to exclude yesterday's feelings and concentrate only on today's feelings in each of the life areas. Also, try *not* to allow one category to influence the results of other categories.

	Completely unhappy						Completely happy			
Cannabis use/non-use	1	2	3	4	5	6	7	8	9	10
Alcohol use/non-use	1	2	3	4	5	6	7	8	9	10
Other drug use/non-use	1	2	3	4	5	6	7	8	9	10
Relationship with boyfriend/ girlfriend	1	2	3	4	5	6	7	8	9	10
Relationship with friends	1	2	3	4	5	6	7	8	9	10
Relationship with parents/ caregivers	1	2	3	4	5	6	7	8	9	10
School	1	2	3	4	5	6	7	8	9	10
Social activities	1	2	3	4	5	6	7	8	9	10
Recreational activities	1	2	3	4	5	6	7	8	9	10
Personal habits	1	2	3	4	5	6	7	8	9	10
Legal issues	1	2	3	4	5	6	7	8	9	10
Money management	1	2	3	4	5	6	7	8	9	10
Emotional life (feelings)	1	2	3	4	5	6	7	8	9	10
Communication	1	2	3	4	5	6	7	8	9	10
General happiness	1	2	3	4	5	6	7	8	9	10
Other _____	1	2	3	4	5	6	7	8	9	10

Note: Based on Meyers and Smith[7]

The Goals of Counselling

The Happiness Scale forms the basis for the Goals of Counselling. Each of the areas listed on the Happiness Scale are included in the Goals of Counselling form. According to ACRA, there are two main aims of the Goals of Counselling procedure:

1 to help the young person develop specific goals relating to each area
2 to work out action plans relating to those goals.

As you'll see later, the Goals of Counselling worksheet allows for these aims to be achieved. It gives a solid framework with which we can identify goals, and plan for their achievement. Meyers[6] cautions us to help our clients set short-term goals. We are not aiming for the end of the rainbow in session one. During ACRA training, workers are encouraged to bear Box 10.5 in mind when it comes to the goals of counselling.

BOX 10.5 The Goals of Counselling[6]

- Ensure the worksheet contains the same life areas as the Happiness Scale.
- Don't try to address everything at once; help the adolescent choose a category to work on.
- Set short-term goals that are scheduled to be completed in the near future.
- Have a step-by-step overall strategy for attaining chosen goals.
- Explore and address any obstacles that may get in the way.
- Assign homework for each week.

When planning goals with teenagers, ensure the tasks you set together are ones that can realistically be completed in the allocated time frame. Make the task something that is in the adolescent's control. If the plan is dependent on an external person, there is the risk that the other person may not be available. SMART planning is a mnemonic drawn from business that can be helpful when devising a strategy with clients.[8] Essentially, a plan should be Specific, Measurable, Assignable, Realistic and Timed.

Remember if you set homework tasks with a client, it is *vital* that you review it at the start of the next session. Consider how demotivating it would be for a teenager who has gone to the effort of following through on their practice exercises if they aren't given the opportunity to share them. Likewise, it's important to check that the client is at least trying to complete the plan. Spend the initial part of the session discussing the previous week's homework exercises.

Explore how the adolescent got on with the task. Identify what went well, what didn't work out and what obstacles they encountered. Address difficulties

Sample Goals of Counselling worksheet

Name: _____ Date: _____

Problem areas/goals *'In the area of _____ I would like:'*	Intervention	Time frame
1 Marijuana use/non-use		
2 Alcohol use/non-use		
3 Other drug use/non-use		
4 Relationship with boyfriend/girlfriend		
5 Relationship with friends		
6 Relationship with parents/caregivers		
7 School		
8 Social activities		
9 Recreational activities		
10 Personal habits		
11 Legal issues		
12 Money management		
13 Emotional life (my feelings)		
14 Communication		
15 General happiness		
16 Other		

_____ (Participant signature)   _____ (Date)

_____ (Counsellor signature)   _____ (Date)

Note: Based on Meyers and Smith[7]

and reinforce strengths. Remember if a plan doesn't work out, it was the plan, not the person that failed. Be ready to re-evaluate, re-plan and reinforce.

An outline of other Adolescent Community Reinforcement Approach procedures

Relapse prevention

Relapse can be part of the process when adolescents are making changes in their substance use. ACRA teaches therapists a specific way in which to work with it. After a relapse, a new FA is conducted, specific to the recent use. This helps to identify relapse-prone areas or high-risk situations. This allows the young person to develop an 'early warning system' and ultimately 'interrupt a chain of events leading to relapse'.

Case example

- Sinead has a fight with her boyfriend when he cancels a date
- She worries he's cheating on her
- She feels upset and angry
- She ignores her mother's attempts to talk to her
- She storms out of the house
- She walks through the park where she used to use drugs with her friends
- She sees her old using buddies sitting around a small fire
- She smells the weed they're smoking
- She walks over 'to say hello'
- She sits down and takes a drag of a joint when it's offered to her

---

In the case example given here, the worker would help the adolescent map out the chain of events and would encourage her to reflect on the various choices she made. For example, the professional might ask, 'tell me about the decision to leave the house?' If you were to use the analogy of a bus journey with a final stop of using drugs, you ask the client to reflect on where they might have gotten off the bus. Ultimately, the goal of reviewing the chain of events is to heighten awareness and encourage the adolescent to reflect on what they're doing. Relapses don't just happen and this new awareness can empower clients and help them plan to make different choices in the future.

Problem-solving protocol

In this procedure, the professional's goal is to teach the young person a way of approaching problems. While you might choose one problem to work on, the procedure itself, once taught and applied, can become part of the adolescent's new coping skills set. Meyers[6] suggests the following eight steps.

1 Create a narrow, focused definition of the problem; our job is to help the adolescent identify a specific and manageable problem to focus on.

2 Spend time teasing out possible solutions. These should ideally come from the client. We don't knock any solutions; rather, we elicit as many options as possible.

3 Then comes the task of eliminating any unwanted ones. The client is asked to identify which ones don't seem realistic, doable or desired.

4 Now we work with the adolescent to identify one potential solution and explore, in a step-by-step manner, how the client envisions using this solution.

5 An exploration of possible obstacles then occurs. What might get in the way of this potential solution? Are there any stumbling blocks? Pitfalls?

6 For every possible obstacle, we work with the adolescent to address it. If the obstacle appears insurmountable, then it's time to pick a different solution.

7 Once a solution is established, and possible obstacles are addressed, we get down to the business of assigning a specific task (remember your SMART planning).

8 Finally, at the next session, we spend some time evaluating the outcome. How did the adolescent get on with his or her task? What was done? What was the outcome? Does the solution need to be modified? Were there any unforeseen obstacles?

It's helpful to use the ACRA problem-solving steps when undertaking this process with a client. Copies of these are available in Meyers and Smith's book *A Clinical Guide to Alcohol Treatment*[7] and in the Cannabis Youth Treatment Series manual.[5]

Sobriety sampling

Referred to as the 'acid test' relating to suitability for outpatient treatment, this procedure encourages the building of an adolescent's confidence in his or her ability to remain sober. Essentially, it's presented as taking 'time out' from drinking or using so that the adolescent can see what it's like, hence the name sampling. The counsellor works with the adolescent to negotiate a period whereby he or she agrees not to drink/use. If the adolescent agrees to this procedure, a detailed plan needs to be developed for the agreed time frame. The therapist and client work together to identify high-risk situations for relapse and a plan is drawn up for how the client plans to deal with these relapse-prone areas.

CONCLUSION

ACRA offers professionals a clear framework for working with young substance users. The procedures are evidence-based and promote empowerment, choice and awareness that reinforcement doesn't have to come from a bottle, syringe or tray of tablets. Homework is an essential part of the process and empowers clients. We are not the experts on their lives, they are. The supportive, problem-solving, psycho-educational components to this model make it one that has real power to effect change.

Training in the Adolescent Community Reinforcement Approach

While it is impossible to cover all areas of this model in this chapter, it's worth noting that Meyers travels the world to train professionals in this counselling approach. The training programme consists of 2.5 days of training, followed by a clinical practice period during which trainees submit taped sessions of their work with clients. Further details of his worldwide training schedule are available online (www.robertjmeyersphd.com).

FURTHER READING

➡ Smith JE, Meyers RJ. *Motivating Substance Abusers to Enter Treatment: working with family members.* New York, NY: Guilford Press; 2004.

REFERENCES

1 Heather N, Robertson I. *Problem Drinking.* 3rd ed. Oxford: Oxford Medical Publications; 1997.
2 Siegal S. Drug anticipation and drug addiction: the 1998 h. David Archibald lecture. *Addiction.* 1999; **94**(8): 1113–14.
3 Meyers RJ, Miller WR. *A Community Reinforcement Approach to Addiction Treatment.* New York, NY: Cambridge University Press; 2006.
4 Clark D. Conditioning models of addiction: part 1. *Drink Drug News.* 9 October 2006: 15. Available at: http://drinkanddrugsnews.com/wp-content/uploads/2013/07/DDN091006.pdf (accessed 13 August 2013).
5 Godley SH, Meyers RJ, Smith JE, *et al. The Adolescent Community Reinforcement Approach for Adolescent Cannabis Users, Cannabis Youth Treatment (CYT) Series.* Vol. 4. DHHS Pub. No. 01–3489. Rockville MD: Center for Substance Abuse Treatment; Substance Abuse and Mental Health Services Administration; 2001.
6 Meyers RJ; Blanchardstown Local Drug Task Force. *Training Manual: Adolescent Community Reinforcement Approach (ACRA).* Dublin: Blanchardstown Local Drug Task Force; 2011.
7 Meyers RJ, Smith JE. *A Clinical Guide to Alcohol Treatment: the community reinforcement approach.* New York, NY: Guilford Press; 1995.
8 Doran GT. There's a S.M.A.R.T. way to write management's goals and objectives. *Manage Rev.* 1981; **70**(11): 35–6.

CHAPTER 11

Other treatment approaches

In previous chapters we explored interventions for substance misuse including the Adolescent Community Reinforcement Approach and Motivational Interviewing. These are interventions with collaborative and cognitive behavioural underpinnings. In this chapter, systemic approaches, 12-step models, self-help groups and therapeutic communities (TCs) are examined. We discuss the use of contingency management (CM) and medication, and while not stand-alone treatments, there is evidence they can be useful adjuncts to therapeutic programmes. Finally, the strengths and weaknesses of drug screening are presented.

SYSTEMIC OR FAMILY-FOCUSED THERAPEUTIC INTERVENTIONS

A number of family-based models have been manualised that are effective in responding to substance-abusing adolescents.[1] A recent meta-analysis indicates that family-based interventions yield superior outcomes to individual approaches.[2] All require the therapist to engage in an active and substantial manner with immediate family or carers and with people and organisations connected with the teen. They are strengths focused, as are many of the individual therapy approaches.

Multidimensional Family Therapy

Multidimensional Family Therapy (MDFT) was developed by Howard Liddle and, somewhat uniquely, specifically with substance use in mind. It is *not* an adaptation of an adult-based programme. It is a highly regarded treatment and has been comprehensively evaluated.[3,4]

MDFT, an outpatient clinic treatment, focuses on adolescents and their families. Importantly, the therapist is encouraged to proactively seek to engage with the wider system around the family, by phone and in person. This may include criminal justice, education and social care systems. Over a time of engagement, attention is devoted to the adolescent's functioning, family management, the parent–adolescent relationship and parenting skills. MDFT has been studied with other adolescent-focused outpatient treatment approaches in the large Cannabis Youth Treatment study.[5] It compared very favourably with alternative treatment models in well-designed studies.[2] While MDFT gives similar outcomes to individual-focused adolescent approaches after treatment and in the early months following treatment, it delivers superior outcomes a year later.[6,7]

It is an intense intervention with sessions offered between one and three times a week over a period of 3–6 months. As a package, it is more expensive than the more individual-focused treatments such as the Adolescent Community Reinforcement Approach. MDFT sessions can occur both in an outpatient clinic setting and/or in the client's home. It is tailored to the individual needs of the adolescent and his or her family.

Training in MDFT does not require the therapist to have any previous experience or qualifications in family therapy but it is intensive. There are three stages a professional can potentially progress through.[8] First is to be a *therapist*, next a *supervisor* and finally some supervisors opt to train as a *trainer*. In order to be certified as a therapist, individuals must complete a 6- to 7-month intensive training that includes several on-site training sessions delivered by a MDFT trainer. It also involves ongoing case consultation via telephone once or twice a week, review of real-life audiovisual sessions and written examinations and case reports.

Functional Family Therapy

Functional Family Therapy (FFT) was initially developed by James Alexander and colleagues at the University of Utah.[9] FFT initially focused on serious conduct problems and antisocial behaviour in adolescence. One of the key philosophies of the approach is to work with families' strengths to achieve small changes. There is a goal of assisting them to accomplish the tasks most relevant *to their specific family*, and to use strategies that fit best for *themselves*. FFT has been evaluated and numerous research publications highlight the positive outcomes it achieves with adolescent substance users.[1,10]

FFT is a relatively short-term intervention, typically lasting 12 sessions. Sessions are delivered both in an outpatient setting and in the family's home but can occur in other locations such as in criminal justice facilities, mental health clinics or schools. The therapist seeks to identify what is working well within a family and builds upon this. In terms of the clinical and treatment process, there are five identified phases that occur after a pre-treatment period. Therapists are encouraged to obtain repeated and constant feedback from the families throughout their engagement.[9]

Multisystemic Therapy

Multisystemic Therapy (MST) was developed by Scott Henggler and was initially developed to focus exclusively on dealing with juvenile criminal behaviour.[11] It is an intensive treatment with therapists typically meeting with the family many times each week. The therapist is required to acquire an excellent understanding of the teen's context. This requires meetings in the family home, the school or vocational setting and also in more informal settings such as where the adolescent 'hangs out'. MST is responsive to crises that occur for the teenager and his or her family. The team of therapists are on call 24 hours a day. Naturally, a single therapist cannot support such an intensive intervention alone. A team of therapists needs to be trained in order to roll it out.

The goals of MST are to:

- increase parenting skills
- improve relationships within the family
- build connections between the teen and friends who are not involved in substance use
- improve academic or vocational performance
- assist the adolescent's involvement in prosocial activities such as sport or youth groups
- draw in additional support from the wider family, neighbours and the community.

12-STEP MODELS

Alcoholics Anonymous (AA) and Narcotics Anonymous (NA) are worldwide self-help groups that are based on the idea that addiction is a disease for which there is no known cure. However, recovery is possible, if affected individuals follow the 12-Step programme.

12-Step fellowships

Bill Wilson, a stockbroker who had self-reported chronic alcoholism, founded the AA fellowship in 1935. He sought spiritual support for his alcoholism in the Oxford Group, a religious programme. It is from this that he developed AA. In the past 8 decades, the 12 steps have been applied to numerous problems, and there are millions of members in these groups worldwide.

AA, NA and many other 'anonymous' programmes are based on the idea that people need to admit they are powerless over alcohol (or another substance/problem) and that their lives are no longer manageable. New members attend daily for the first 90 days, and continue to attend regularly for the rest of their lives. Members identify themselves as 'addicts' or 'alcoholics' and the programme contends that attendance at meetings and working the programme is how members recover. Meetings all over the world follow a similar format. A secretary opens the meeting, asking various members to read passages from the *Big Book of AA* or the *Basic Text of NA*. Following this, one member, who has a level of 'clean time' will act as 'chair' and tell the story of his or her journey into substance misuse, his or her discovery of the 12-step programme and how life has changed since joining. Instillation of hope and a sense of identification are benefits of this approach.

Central to the programme are the steps themselves. Attendance at meetings is promoted, but the programme involves working through the steps in sequence with a 12-step sponsor. There are fellowship approved 12-step guides that contain questions that the member answers and shares with their sponsor. Questions in the first step may include the following.

- How has my disease affected my life: physically? mentally? spiritually? emotionally?
- Describe times when I have tried to stop and failed?
- Describe times when I have tried (and failed) to control my drinking/using?
- What have I neglected because of my use of drugs/alcohol?

They are asked to share this information with other group members. It is expected that members cease use of all substances of misuse. For example, if someone attends NA with a cocaine problem, he or she is expected to also stop using other drugs and alcohol.

Each step has a guiding 'spiritual principle' such as honesty, willingness, trust or forgiveness, and the overall tenet is that through working the steps, the person can have a spiritual awakening. For some, the use of words like 'spirituality' and 'higher power' along with the appearance of the word 'God' in the steps can be off-putting. Nevertheless, the programme is applicable to those with no religious beliefs. The 'power greater' can be the group itself.

A 2009 Cochrane Review of AA found that 'AA may help patients to accept treatment and keep patients in treatment more than alternative treatments.'[14] However, this finding was not conclusive. Empirical research has only been conducted recently on the 12 steps and there is much more to be done. Importantly, research conducted with members will probably not include the views of those who found the programme unhelpful.

When considering adolescents, we need to be mindful of the fact that 12-step programmes are not monitored and the majority of members are older, often with far more protracted histories of substance use. One way around this is for the AA/NA helpline to be contacted prior to initial attendance. Often, long-term members, with substantial sobriety, are willing to meet with and bring a new member to their first meeting. In some areas, there are meetings specifically for young people.

AA, NA and CA (Cocaine Anonymous) offer open meetings, where the public can attend but not participate. For professionals who are unfamiliar with the programme, we recommend attending one before you provide clients with a meeting list.

There is a substantial divide in the professional substance misuse field between proponents of the 12-step or disease model and other models. This is a pity, as they all have strengths and limitations. What works for one person may not work for another. As professionals, it is useful and appropriate to have an awareness of as many potential supports as possible. Twelve-step groups are a useful and supportive way of encouraging behaviour change. However, they are not, as they often claim, the only way.

12-Step facilitation

Substance Abuse and Mental Health Services Administration's National Registry of Evidence-Based Programs and Practices defines 12-step facilitation as a 'structured, and manual-driven approach to facilitating early recovery from alcohol abuse, alcoholism, and other drug abuse and addiction problems.'[12] It is a brief (12- to 15-session) manualised way of working with clients who have substance misuse problems. There are two main goals:

1 acceptance of the necessity for abstinence
2 willingness to attend and participate in 12-step meetings such as AA or NA, as a way of 'staying clean or sober'.

The US National Institute on Alcohol Abuse and Alcoholism produced a 12-step facilitation manual as part of the Project Match study.[13] Project Match was a large controlled study of various treatments with alcohol-dependent adults. It clearly states that the fellowships, and not the therapists, are the primary vehicle for change. The role of the therapist is to introduce the client to the concepts of AA/NA and to prepare them for involvement in the fellowships. In the opening sessions, the therapist builds rapport, encourages participation in the process and explains the AA understanding of addiction. The therapist works with the client to obtain a substance use history that includes reflection on antecedents and consequences to use. In subsequent sessions, the therapist will teach the client how the fellowships work, help them understand key concepts such as 'surrender', and promote involvement in AA/NA. Clients' homework involves reading, journaling and attending meetings.[13] Some adolescent substance treatment programmes, particularly residential ones, adhere to the 12-step model.

OTHER PEER-LED SELF-HELP PROGRAMMES: LIFERING

Other group-based self-help approaches have emerged with the realisation that the 12-step approach does not work for everyone. LifeRing was developed in 1999 in California. Segregation by 'substance of choice' does *not* occur, with those using alcohol attending the same meeting as those dependent on other drugs.

Core elements of LifeRing include the '3-S Philosophy'. This stands for:

- *Sobriety*: the *goal* of abstinence from all non-prescribed psychoactive drugs is necessary.
- *Secularity*: LifeRing is not an atheist-agnostic organisation; there is peaceful coexistence and respect for participants from all faiths and those with none; meetings seek to create an atmosphere of empathy, concern, care, love and respect.
- *Self-help*: participants are expected to take personal responsibility for their own recovery and, unlike 12-step models, do not encourage members to hand themselves over to God or a Higher Power.

The motto of LifeRing is 'empower your sober self'. They conceptualise that within the substance-dependent person, especially at the time of treatment seeking, there is a conflict between the *addicted self* and the *sober self*. If people with addictions focus their relationships on obtaining, using and talking about the substance, the addicted self will overpower any nascent sober self. However, if people focus on their sober selves, this can ultimately 'shrink' the addicted self. Participants focus on the benefits of sobriety and the challenges they may face in coming weeks. Participants are encouraged to determine and adhere to their *own* personal recovery plan. Perhaps if there is a fundamental difference between 12-step approaches and LifeRing, it is that in AA/NA, people are actively encouraged to dwell upon the negative while in LifeRing, they are encouraged to dwell upon the positive.

Self-help groups such as AA or LifeRing can form an important component of a teenager's treatment, commencing alongside and then continuing long after an episode of professionally delivered treatment. While LifeRing is a relatively new organisation its structures and philosophies provide a better fit than AA or NA for adolescents who have participated in a substance abuse treatment programme utilising cognitive behavioural therapy, Motivational Interviewing or solution-focused approaches. However, like 12 Step, the effectiveness of LifeRing with adolescents has not been scientifically evaluated. Other group formats are available including SMART recovery, but they are outside the scope of this book.

THERAPEUTIC COMMUNITIES

The early therapeutic communities

Synanon, the first TC for substance users, was founded by Charles 'Chuck' Dederich in California in 1958.[15] The very name 'therapeutic community' implies one of the main tenets: being part of the community is therapeutic. The central goal of TCs is to help clients stay clean, and they believe in abstinence. Historically, the belief was that only when the client's defences and drug identity was broken down, could they be built up into a productive member of society. They were facilitated to do this by others with experience of substance misuse problems.

The evolution of therapeutic communities

According to the Center for Substance Abuse Treatment's *The Therapeutic Community Curriculum Trainer's Manual*,[16] TCs have evolved in the following ways.

- There is a mix of professionals that consists of trained therapists with no history of substance use, as well as recovering people who have gone through a TC *and* professional training.
- TCs have adopted evidence-based practice and include evaluation and outcome studies.
- There are requirements regarding standards, training and qualifications of staff, and TCs have set up worldwide professional organisations.
- There are 14 common programme components that define the TC approach.
- The approach has been adapted for special populations (e.g. adolescents, women) and special settings (e.g. prisons).

While TCs are no longer the 3-year programmes they once were, treatment can still take 18 months. Participants work their way through a programme involving behaviour therapy principles. Good behaviour is rewarded and privileges are lost when clients don't engage appropriately. Participants engage in a range of therapeutic activities throughout the day. According to the US National Institute on Drug Abuse's research report on TCs, the TC day starts at 7 a.m. and ends at 11 p.m.[17] Activities include:

- house meetings
- clinical groups
- encounter groups
- vocational work
- educational activities
- community activities
- concept groups.

Clients learn TC concepts and practise these until they are internalised. Psycho-educational components are included, with clients attending lectures on topics like relapse prevention, changing negative thoughts and goal-setting. There are still groups where people are encouraged to 'encounter' their pain, secrets and shadow side. TCs have their own jargon, which clients and staff are encouraged to use.

Therapeutic communities adapted for adolescents

TCs specific to adolescents have been developed in some countries. Research tells us that adolescents who enter TCs have 'serious substance use and behaviour problems that render them dysfunctional in many areas.'[18] TCs adapted for adolescents have a number of differences, such as:

- shorter treatment duration
- treatment progresses along developmental dimensions
- less confrontational
- more staff supervision
- assessment for other disorders
- less emphasis on vocational strategies, and inclusion of more educational interventions (e.g. school work)
- more family involvement
- inclusion of recreational activities.

While long, intense programmes are not for everyone, they have evidenced success. One 2000 study found 'there were significant reductions in drug use and criminal activity, and the most consistent predictors of positive outcomes were completion of treatment and not associating with deviant peers posttreatment.'[18] Once again we note different treatments work for different teenagers.

CONTINGENCY MANAGEMENT

In recent years, CM has emerged as a new behavioural treatment approach – it is mostly used as an adjunct to other treatments.[19] Research to date has focused mainly on cocaine-dependent adults. It is controversial. Many clinicians and members of the public are opposed to giving drug users financial or other rewards for ceasing drug use.

In CM, the client obtains tangible positive reinforcers (rewards) for objective behaviour change. For example, they receive a shopping voucher for provision of a urine sample that screens negative for drugs. The positive effects of CM have been unambiguously demonstrated when compared to traditional treatments.[20] Research indicates it can support adherence to other elements of treatment and improves treatment retention. There are some concerns that there is frequent rapid relapse following cessation and it can be expensive to operate. Most evaluated CM programmes use escalating rewards for increasing lengths of abstinence. If an individual lapses, the reward magnitude reverts to baseline once again. As with any positive reinforcement schedule, frequent and prompt reinforcement works best.

While most research on CM has occurred in adults, there are good reasons to think that it will also work in adolescents.[21] Unlike adults, adolescents in treatment are less intrinsically motivated. They tend to access treatment because *others* are concerned. CM can partially compensate for this by providing an additional external reinforcer. Research provides evidence of its positive impact in adolescent cannabis use as an adjunct to a treatment programme involving Motivational Interviewing, cognitive behavioural therapy and substantial parent input.[20] Parents were directly involved in elements of the CM programme by identifying and implementing 'rewards' for abstinence via praise and provision of treats such as going to the cinema. CM has also been used to good effect in adolescent smoking cessation. Further research is needed to better understand this intervention and its role with adolescents.

MEDICATION IN THE TREATMENT OF TEENAGE SUBSTANCE USE

The mainstay of treatment with adolescents is psychosocial in nature. The role for medication is very limited. In situations where medications are used, this should *always* occur alongside simultaneous psychosocial interventions. Indeed, even in the adult age-range, despite intensive investigation and investment by pharmaceutical companies in recent decades, there are *relatively few* agents that have a prominent role in the treatment of substance dependence. A comprehensive review of use of medication in adolescent substance use disorders is available at the National Treatment Agency in the UK.[22]

Medications used to treat adolescent substance use fall into three main categories, considered here. There are agents that assist detoxification, relapse prevention and medications used for substitution treatment.

Detoxification

A number of substances can cause physiological dependence – most commonly alcohol, benzodiazepines and opiates. People who consume these drugs on a daily basis over a sustained period of time, experience specific withdrawal symptoms upon sudden cessation. Withdrawal symptoms include sweating, tremor, restlessness, insomnia and irritability. Scales have been developed to monitor withdrawal symptoms from alcohol (the Clinical Institute Withdrawal Assessment for Alcohol scale, or CIWA-Ar) and opiates (Objective Opioid Withdrawal Scale [OOWS] and the Subjective Opioid Withdrawal Scale

[SOWS]).[23,24] The goal of a medical detoxification is to minimise withdrawal symptoms and reduce the occurrence of withdrawal complications.

Before discussing individual treatments it is worth considering the entire concept of detoxification, often called a detox. Contrary to popular belief, *detoxification is not a treatment of addiction*. Substance-using behaviour is to some extent perpetuated by the presence of withdrawal symptoms, with the dependent individual continuing to use the substance in order to stop their 'withdrawal sickness'. These symptoms act as negative reinforcers of sustained substance use. In other words, when someone who is dependent stops using, they are punished with withdrawal symptoms. They are then rewarded with the removal of these symptoms when they recommence using. In truth, there are a huge number of other psychosocial factors that perpetuate ongoing substance use. Consequently, it is pointless to embark on a detoxification intervention if the psychosocial factors are not addressed.

Historically, people who were alcohol or heroin dependent were admitted to hospital, provided with a simple detox and then sent on their way. Almost inevitably, the majority rapidly returned to substance use. The relapse rates following simple outpatient detoxification are in excess of 90%. If a person has built their entire social life around drinking behaviour, it is naive to expect that the provision of a simple detox will cause them to cease alcohol use. Typically, when such a person completes their detox and returns to their social environment they will drift back into the previously established behaviour. Consequently, it is our advice that detoxification should only be considered as part of a broader psychosocial intervention. The key question that must be asked by the client, their family and those drawing up the treatment plan is, 'what is the likelihood of abstinence being sustained following detoxification?' If the answer to this question is 'very unlikely' then further work needs to be undertaken in order to build on the coping skills or other supports to assist them in avoiding relapse. It is our view that detoxification should be one of the last steps taken in provision of treatment for someone who is physically dependent on a substance and *not rushed into as the initial step.*

Provision of a detox-based intervention to an individual with little hope of a positive outcome is a potentially dangerous thing to do. First, the experience of rapid relapse following detox can cause patient, family and therapeutic staff to become hopeless about the individual's ability to make and sustain positive change. Secondly, there is emerging evidence that repeated experience of withdrawal symptoms and detox episodes linked to severe alcohol dependence can be associated with increased progression of the neurocognitive damage associated with alcohol dependence.[25] An ill-planned opiate detox is potentially more dangerous, as the individual's tolerance to opiates will fall rapidly as he or she detoxes. If the individual then returns to heroin use in the following days or weeks, there is very high risk of an accidental overdose due to reduced tolerance and this can be fatal.

Alcohol detox

Thankfully in adolescence, physiological dependence on alcohol is relatively uncommon. Adolescent alcohol use often follows a binge pattern where alcohol is consumed on a daily basis for a number of days followed by a break. Irish adolescents are among the heaviest drinkers in Europe. Within a catchment area of over 300 000 people, we have not found it necessary to commence any adolescent on an alcohol detox in our clinical service over the past five years even though alcohol is the primary substance misused in 25% of the teenagers who attend.

Where an adolescent does report a clear history of withdrawal symptoms associated with their alcohol use, a detox can be considered. For most adolescents this can be safely conducted on an outpatient basis using the benzodiazepine, chlordiazepoxide (Librium). This medication can only be initiated under medical supervision and detox will occur over 5–7 days. While rare in adolescents, withdrawal epileptic seizures are worthy of consideration. If a person exhibits severe withdrawal symptoms or has a history of past seizures during withdrawals, medical admission for detoxification should be strongly considered.

The most dangerous type of alcohol withdrawals result in delirium tremens (DTs), but this complication is rare, especially in adolescents. It is characterised by delirium (i.e. an acute confusional state) accompanied by severe abnormalities in blood pressure and pulse rate, vivid hallucinations, global confusion, tremor, fumbling movements of the hands, insomnia, and other physical and neurologic symptoms. It typically has its onset 2–4 days after cessation of drinking. While older studies of DTs reported a mortality of up to 20%, with modern treatment mortality is closer to 1%. Patient characteristics associated with increased risk of DTs included past history of DTs, age over 40 years, a history of withdrawal seizures and current medical illness (e.g. pneumonia).

Benzodiazepine detox

Again, in our experience benzodiazepine misuse in adolescence tends to follow a binge pattern with use of large numbers of tablets on a daily basis for a short number of days followed by periods of abstinence also lasting a number of days. However, where a teen reports daily use, with physical withdrawal symptoms, a detox could be contemplated. Benzodiazepine detox occurs over a much longer period than alcohol detox. If a person has been on substantial quantities of benzodiazepines over a period of months or years, the standard outpatient approach to detox would last weeks. One serious problem with prescribing an outpatient benzodiazepine detox is that it is difficult to monitor adherence. Even if the teenager attends the clinic on a daily basis to pick up their medication, they will have to take this in divided doses later in the day and before going to sleep. This requires a degree of parental supervision. It is also difficult to monitor whether or not the teenager is 'topping up' the prescribed medication with tablets obtained on the street or from another doctor. For these reasons, it is our recommendation that the small number of adolescents who require a benzodiazepine detox should receive this in a residential setting.

Opiate detox

While opiate withdrawals are physically unpleasant, they are not as dangerous as alcohol withdrawals. Opiate withdrawal symptoms tend to mimic those of 'the flu'. Two broad categories of medication can be used to assist in opiate detox. The first option is to use other opiate drugs such as methadone or buprenorphine, which are long-acting medications. A typical opiate detox occurs over 10–21 days.

One danger of methadone, most often used in detox, is that it has a powerful opiate effect itself. If the dose is increased too quickly or the doctor overestimates the degree of physical dependence, they may cause an opiate overdose for that adolescent. This can have fatal outcomes. Consequently, only doctors who have obtained substantial training in the treatment of opiate dependence should initiate methadone. Substantial daily monitoring of the adolescent should be conducted in the context of a multidisciplinary psychosocial intervention.

The alternative option is to use medication such as lofexidene. This drug is not an opiate but instead acts on a different neurotransmitter system (noradrenaline). Taking lofexidene reduces withdrawal symptoms. Medication must be taken three to four times daily. Consequently, the adolescent will need to be supervised either by family or professionals, or possibly have treatment delivered in a residential setting. As lofexedine is not as effective as methadone at managing withdrawal symptoms, dropout from treatment is more likely.

Medication use in managing withdrawals from stimulant drugs and cannabis

The withdrawal syndromes associated with sudden cessation of stimulants and cannabis is associated with few objective physical problems. However, it has become clear that there are psychological withdrawal symptoms following periods of sustained and heavy use. Withdrawal symptoms typically include irritability, low mood, restlessness and poor sleep.[26,27] There are no agonist drugs which can be prescribed. Symptoms should be managed with psychosocial interventions and judicious use of adjunctive medications to target specific symptoms.

Insomnia can be a frustrating symptom for clients.[27] Sleep problems may be compounded by a poor sleep routine during the weeks and months of regular drug use. Substance-dependent youth may present with evidence of sleep reversal, typically staying up late at night and sleeping much of the day. The core strategy to manage such sleep difficulties is the introduction of better sleeping habits. Sleeping during the day should be discouraged. Consideration can be given to prescribing hypnotics such as zoplicone for a limited period. However, such drugs are sedating. They require monitoring as they may interact with other medication prescribed as part of the detox. This can result in excessive sedation and possibly overdose. Also, in light of the real concerns regarding the misuse potential of hypnotic medications, prescribing should probably be reserved to the residential setting or supervised closely by an adult caregiver.

Medication used in maintenance or substitution treatment

While maintenance or substitution treatment tend to be unpopular among the general public and many politicians, some of these treatments have significant evidence to back up their use in adults. The most established maintenance treatment is that of ongoing methadone provision to people who are opioid dependent. There is now a vast literature which indicates that heroin-dependent adults who receive methadone maintenance treatment demonstrate reduced heroin use, reduced rates of unsafe injecting behaviours, improved psychological well-being and social functioning.[24] Nevertheless, many people, including professionals involved in substance use treatment, are uncomfortable with the idea of providing people who have problematic drug use with a similar drug. They view it as substituting one problem for another. The core issue with methadone maintenance is that *it does nothing* to tackle the individual's *physical* dependence on opiates.

While there is significant evidence for the value of methadone maintenance treatment in adults, this intervention has undergone little evaluation in adolescents. Indeed, in many countries it is not possible to prescribe a substitution treatment to a person under the age of 18. However, the limited evidence indicates that adolescents who are prescribed methadone do make significant progress.[28]

During the 1990s, Ireland had the youngest population of treatment-seeking heroin users in Europe, where the standard treatment provision was methadone maintenance. This treatment was also provided to adolescents. The outcome for these adolescents has been partially evaluated and indicated reduced heroin use.[28] There is also evidence to indicate reduced unsafe injecting behaviour in that the incidence of hepatitis C infection was lower than that seen in those offered detox-type treatments. Despite this and other evidence of the potential usefulness of methadone maintenance treatments in the most severely heroin-dependent adolescents, it remains controversial. Again, it is essential that it is delivered in the context of a multidisciplinary treatment intervention that focuses broadly on the adolescent's psychosocial functioning and actively works with family to support major changes in the adolescent's lifestyle.[22]

Buprenorphine has emerged as a viable alternative to methadone.[24] It has a longer half-life and a lower risk of overdose, but it is more expensive. It may also be easier to detox off buprenorphine than methadone. For these reasons, some suggest it should be the first-line treatment for opioid-dependent adolescents. Induction onto buprenorphine requires planning and, if done inappropriately, it can bring on significant withdrawal symptoms, which may deter the client from persisting with treatment.[25]

Medications to assist in relapse prevention

Disulfiram (Antabuse)

Disulfiram is an aversive treatment used to deal with alcohol dependence for decades. The vast majority of research has occurred with adults though some has looked at its usefulness in adolescents.[23]

This medication interferes with the metabolic breakdown of alcohol in the liver. This causes a build-up of the chemical acetaldehyde, which results in a number of unpleasant symptoms including severe nausea if alcohol is consumed. It is prescribed to some patients who are abstinent from alcohol and who are keen to maintain abstinence. If they do have a slip, the extremely unpleasant physical symptoms act as a negative reinforcer of abstinence behaviour.

While certainly not part of a standard treatment of alcohol-dependent adolescents, it can have a role in some cases for motivated teens, particularly if there is active and ongoing support by family or caregivers. Ideally, daily supervision of this medication will be monitored and supervised by a parent. Many individuals report getting cravings to use a drug they are trying to give up and many give in to these cravings. Generally these urges last a short period of time. For a person on disulfiram, they will have to wait for the medication to leave their system before they can drink alcohol without getting sick. By the time this happens the urges have often passed. Interestingly, disulfiram has also been used in the treatment of adult cocaine dependence. There is some evidence that it can have a small, positive effect in this cohort.[25]

Naltrexone

Naltrexone is a medication with an established role in relapse prevention for opioid-dependent individuals. However, it is certainly not a miracle drug. It works by binding to the opiate receptor in the brain. Although it binds very tightly to these receptors, it has no stimulant activity; it just sits there. If a person who takes naltrexone consumes an opioid drug such as heroin, the heroin is unable to bind to the opioid receptor in the brain that is already occupied by the naltrexone. Consequently, the patient experiences no intoxication effects from the heroin.

Again most research with naltrexone has occurred in adults.[25] While initially, there were substantial hopes that it would prove to be an important drug in sustaining abstinence, the results of research trials have been disappointing. Many opt to stop taking the drug quite quickly. There are concerns that naltrexone may cause mood to deteriorate and suicidal behaviour to increase, possibly due to a blocking effect on the natural opioids in the brain. There have also been concerns about increased fatal overdose risk when people stop naltrexone and return to heroin use.

More recently, research has been undertaken to examine the potential role for naltrexone in the treatment of alcohol use disorders.[25] There is some research to indicate that naltrexone results in reduced relapses among adults who are abstinent following an episode of psychosocial treatment. Similarly, there is some evidence that adults who lapse following treatment, may be less likely to progress to a full relapse if they are on naltrexone. In order to improve patient adherence with this medication, there have been efforts to develop longer acting methods of drug delivery. Implants have been developed and there is also an injectable preparation of this drug.

Acamprosate

Acamprosate has been developed as a medication to reduce cravings in people who are alcohol dependent. There is evidence that it has a modest impact on adult alcohol-dependent patients, causing a small reduction in the proportion who relapse.[25] Its role in adolescents is unclear.

Cocaine vaccine

There is ongoing research to develop a cocaine vaccine. In theory, this vaccine will cause the vaccinated person to develop antibodies against cocaine. Therefore, when they consume this drug the antibodies will intercept the chemical before it has a chance to reach the brain and induce any euphoric effect. Consequently, the vaccine could be similar to the impact of naltrexone in heroin users. Unlike naltrexone, however, ongoing adherence will not be an issue, as the person will be left with the antibodies against cocaine on a permanent or near-permanent basis.

A range of other medications have been experimented with as treatments of cocaine dependence, but most have been found to be ineffective.[25] There is currently no role at this time for any medication in the treatment of cocaine dependence in adolescents.

DRUG SCREENING AND TESTING

When working with adolescents, consideration is often given to the possibility of using some form of drug screen as an intervention. The method of drug screen most commonly used is the analysis of a urine sample. Alternative approaches include testing a saliva or blood sample, or even a hair sample.[29]

Urine drug screens

Urine drug screens are the most widely used form of biological screening in both adolescents and adults. Urine samples can be analysed in a laboratory, but there are also on-site testing kits available. This latter method allows the parent or professional to use a 'dipstick' to get immediate evidence of the presence or absence of substances. The test gives information regarding substance use over the past 1–30 days, dependent on the distribution of the drug within the body and the pace at which it is eliminated (*see* Chapter 3). For example, the body excretes cannabis extremely slowly. If a young person has been smoking cannabis on a daily basis and then ceases use, his or her urine may test positive for up to 1 month after having stopped using. In contrast, other drugs such as cocaine, amphetamines and heroin are cleared from the body more rapidly, usually 3–7 days after cessation of daily use. The urine drug screen *provides no information on the quantity of use*. The test will not distinguish between a person who smokes five joints of cannabis daily and another teenager who smokes one joint of cannabis twice a week. Both these adolescents will test positive.

Biological drug testing in the clinic setting

Many treatment services use biological testing, especially urine screens, as a strategy to monitor substance use during treatment. These samples provide *some* objective evidence of progress or otherwise, during treatment and can be useful. First, they provide objective evidence of abstinence. Second, they can be used as an objective basis upon which to base a contingency management programme – for example, the family or the clinic may put in place positive rewards for the teenager linked to this objective evidence of abstinence. Third, in our clinical experience, some young people *request* ongoing urine drug screens because they say it incentivises them to maintain abstinence. Such adolescents report that the knowledge that they are being monitored and getting the repeated positive feedback on their abstinence is something they find supportive. Others report that it helps them to say no to friends when offered drugs because they have the excuse of saying 'I have to do drug tests'.

Another advantage of drug screening is that it can provide the therapist with early evidence of a lapse. While generally adolescents will self-report a lapse, some may be reluctant to do so. They may be wary because of the anticipated reaction by their family or other adults involved in their lives (e.g. social workers or probation officers). Perhaps surprisingly, it has also been our experience that some adolescents are worried about upsetting the therapist when they lapse. As therapists, we take pride in the successes of adolescents who attain and sustain abstinence. Many adolescents notice this. They also enjoy the affirmation they receive regarding the positive changes they make. When they lapse, many are disappointed in themselves. They may feel they have let their family and even their therapist down. Also, some adolescents who have a long-established avoidant coping style may try to convince themselves that they have the lapse under control and they don't need to tell the therapist. In all of these circumstances, it is useful for the therapist to have the objective evidence of the positive drug screen because it provides an opportunity to identify the lapse early in its course. This maximises the likelihood that they can intervene assertively and work to avoid the lapse becoming a full blown relapse. Again, because the adolescent knows that drug screening is ongoing, this appears to assist them in declaring the fact that they have had a lapse before the drug testing is actually completed. Indeed, we have encountered numerous instances where teenagers report a lapse but the subsequent screen tests negative, because of the elimination of the drug. This of course highlights an important limitation of the screening methods; also false negatives do occur. Another important limitation relates to the fact that many substances such as solvents, LSD, synthetic cannabinoids and most of the novel psychoactive substances such as mephedrone, are simply not included in the majority of tests.

Drug screening outside the clinical context

Many non-clinicians are attracted to the idea of conducting drug screens on adolescents. It is our impression that such professionals place excessive emphasis on screening and have a distorted understanding of the value of such monitoring. Situations where drug screening is considered, or sometimes occurs, include the criminal justice, child protection and school settings.

Juvenile justice settings

Courts and probation services place significant, and we believe excessive, emphasis on the results of drug screens. As already outlined, there are many limitations to urine drug screens, particularly the variable half-life of many substances. While the results of drug screening can provide evidence to indicate abstinence, they are of little value in distinguishing between extremely heavy drug use and relatively light use. Consequently, an adolescent who has made major changes in his or her heroin use, for example, reducing use from injecting five bags of heroin every day to smoking just one bag twice a week will demonstrate absolutely no change on a urine screen. If excessive weight is attached to results of urine tests, the court or probation officer may deal with the adolescent in an excessively punitive manner. In such circumstances, adolescents who cannot obtain and sustain abstinence have no incentive to reduce their use at all. Consequently, the intervention can be counterproductive and can have a negative impact on motivation to change.

When treatment services receive requests from agencies such as the criminal justice or child protection systems for treatment reports on adolescents, we recommend that progress of treatment is described across a number of domains such as psychological and social, as well as providing feedback on the progress in tackling substance use. When reporting changes in substance use to the court, we strongly recommend that more information is provided than simply listing results of drug screens. We believe that specific feedback on drug use should include comment on the teenagers' participation in treatment and their self-reported use. Collateral information should be included from family or others regarding frequency and intensity of intoxication, the therapist's observation of intoxication or otherwise during attendance at appointments. The consistency of self-reported substance use and drugs screen results can also be outlined.

School setting

In recent years there has been significant debate regarding the potential role of urine screens in schools. Some suggest that all students be randomly drug screened. Others suggest a more targeted approach where adolescents who have an identified substance use problem be subjected to routine or random screening. There are cultural differences, with greatest enthusiasm for school-based testing in the United States. However, even in the United States most clinicians are opposed to such screening programmes.[30]

Before embarking on drug screening in a school environment, we recommend that consideration be given to what exactly will happen to the adolescent following a negative, or particularly a positive sample. Will they be suspended or possibly expelled? Will they be mandated to attend some sort of treatment until they provide a negative drug screen? Who will give consent to testing? What will happen to a student where a parent refuses consent? Will the student have to declare use of medically prescribed drugs and, if so, does this represent a breach of his or her right to confidentiality?

A report for the Australian National Council on Drugs highlights the many concerns with school-based drug screening.[31] The most commonly abused substance by school-going adolescents is cannabis. As mentioned earlier, it has a particularly long half-life when tested in urine screens. It is possible that adolescents might opt to use another substance, such as amphetamine or cocaine which will leave their system more rapidly, instead of cannabis if there is a likelihood of being drug tested. In other words, the very presence of drug screening might incentivise them to move towards more risky substances. Again, because the results of the urine screen are rather crude, it does nothing to distinguish the very heavy user from the more episodic user. As with any testing regimen, the screen can only give information on the specific battery of drugs, which are part of the particular drug screen used. Many drugs such as LSD are almost impossible to detect on standard screens. With the emergence of a wide range of novel psychoactive substances in recent years, such as synthetic cannabinoids, there are an increasing number of substances that are not tested. Drug screening is not cheap, whether samples are sent to a laboratory or tested on-site; the test kits typically cost close to €10 each. In a large school of 500 students, even if you are only going to test 10% of students, say, six times per year, this will result in a cost of about €3000 per annum. Given the potentially counter-productive impact of such an approach outlined earlier, this level of cost may be difficult to justify.

CONCLUSION

Treatment of adolescent substance use is a complicated endeavour. There are many treatment approaches and philosophies. Each has inherent strengths and weaknesses. Deciding which treatment to choose and the setting in which to deliver it requires considerable thought and expertise. Police, social workers, judges, youth workers and teachers should seek advice from specialists before directing a young person to any particular treatment model. Medication has a small but definite role in treatment of adolescent substance use disorders, but they should be delivered alongside other psychosocial treatments. Detoxification is not a 'stand alone' addiction treatment, although it can be an important step towards recovery. While drug screening has a useful role in treatment settings, it has little utility on its own.

KEY POINTS

- Family-based interventions to treat adolescent substance misuse have been widely researched and provide strongly positive outcomes.
- Engaging with the young person's environment, wider community and other professionals in substance misuse treatment is positively evidenced.
- Self-help approaches, such as AA and NA, along with 12-step facilitation programmes can work for some adolescents.
- While controversial, CM could be effectively utilised more frequently in adolescent treatment programmes.
- Medication has little role in treatment of adolescent substance use disorders. Medical detoxification is rarely required in this age range, as binge patterns of use predominate.

- Opiate substitution treatment appears to have a role in that small minority of adolescents who become heroin dependent, but only as part of a comprehensive multidisciplinary psychosocial intervention.
- Drug screens can be useful as part of treatment, providing some objective evidence of abstinence and giving early indication of any lapse.
- We urge caution in the use of drug screens in other settings. Without good knowledge of the limitations of these screens, they may cause inappropriate levels of reassurance or alarm.

FURTHER READING

- National Treatment Agency for Substance Misuse. *Building Recovery in Communities: substance misuse among young people 2011–12.* London: National Health Service; 2012. Available at: www.nta.nhs.uk/uploads/yp2012vfinal.pdf
- *Functional Family Therapy:* further information can be found on the FFT homepage (www.fftinc.com/index.html).
- *Multisystemic Therapy:* a wealth of information can be obtained on the MST homepage (www.mstservices.com).
- US Substance Abuse and Mental Health Services Administration (SAMHSA). *Twelve Step Facilitation Therapy.* Available at: www.nrepp.samhsa.gov/ViewIntervention. aspx?id=55
- There is a multitude of information available on the 12 steps using a Google search.
- Further information on LifeRing can be found online (www.lifering.org).
- Gilvarry E, Britton J. National Treatment Agency for Substance Misuse. *Guidance for the Pharmacological Management of Substance Misuse among Young People.* London: Department of Health; 2009. Available at: www.nta.nhs.uk/uploads/guidance_for_the_ pharmacological_management_of_substance_misuse_among_young_people_1009. pdf
- Australian National Council on Drugs. *Drug Testing in Schools: evidence, impacts and alternatives.* Canberra: Australian National Council on Drugs; 2007. Available at: www. ancd.org.au/images/PDF/Researchpapers/rp16_drug_testing_in_schools.pdf?phpMyA dmin=rGQ2XkOOsKjMp24r2sFwuVc5ibb

REFERENCES

1 National Institute on Drug Abuse (NIDA). *Principles of Drug Addiction Treatment: a research-based guide.* 3rd ed. Bethesda, MD: NIDA; 2012.
2 Tanner-Smith EE, Wilson SJ, Lipsey MW. The comparative effectiveness of outpatient treatment for adolescent substance abuse: a meta-analysis. *J Subst Abuse Treat.* 2013; 44(2): 145–58.
3 Phan O, Henderson CE, Angelidis, *et al.* European youth care sites serve different populations of adolescents with cannabis use disorder: baseline and referral data from the INCANT trial. *BMC Psychiatry.* 2011; **11**: 110.

4 Hogue A, Liddle HA. Family-based treatment for adolescent substance abuse: controlled trials and new horizons in services research. *J Fam Ther.* 2009; **31**: 126–54.

5 Dennis ML, Godley SH, Diamond G, *et al.* The Cannabis Youth Treatment (CYT) study: main findings from two randomised trials. *J Subst Abuse Treat.* 2004; **27**(3): 197–213.

6 Liddle HA, Rowe CL, Dakof GA, *et al.* Multidimensional Family Therapy for young adolescent substance abuse: twelve-month outcomes of a randomized controlled trial. *J Consult Clin Psychol.* 2009; **77**(1): 12–25.

7 Sherman C. Multidimensional Family Therapy for adolescent drug abuse offers broad, lasting benefits. *NIDA Notes.* 2010; **23**(3): 13–15.

8 Center for Treatment Research on Adolescent Drug Abuse. *Multidimensional Family Therapy (MDFT) Training, Implementation, and Sustainability.* Miami, FL: Center for Treatment Research on Adolescent Drug Abuse; 2010. Available at: www.med.miami.edu/CTRADA/documents/DescriptionOfMDFTTrainingProgram2011-2012.doc (accessed 13 February 2013).

9 Sexton TL. *Family Therapy in Clinical Practice: an evidence-based treatment model for at risk adolescents.* New York, NY: Routledge; 2011.

10 Waldron HB, Turner CW. Evidence-based psychosocial treatments for adolescent abuser: a review and meta-analysis. *J Clin Child Adolesc Psychol.* 2008; **37**(1): 238–61.

11 Henggeler SW, Halliday-Boykins CA, Cunningham PB, *et al.* Juvenile drug court: enhancing outcomes by integrating evidence-based treatments. *J Consult Clin Psychol.* 2006; **74**(1): 42–54.

12 Substance Abuse and Mental Health Services Administration (SAMHSA). *Twelve Step Facilitation Therapy.* SAMHSA's National Registry of Evidence-based Programmes and Practices. Available at: www.nrepp.samhsa.gov/ViewIntervention.aspx?id=55 (accessed 9 August 2013).

13 Nowinski J, Baker S, Carroll K. *Twelve Step Facilitation Manual: a clinical treatment manual for therapists treating individuals with alcohol abuse and dependence.* National Institute on Alcohol Abuse and Alcoholism. Project Match Monograph Series. Vol. 1. Rockville, MD: National Institute on Alcohol Abuse and Alcoholism; 1992.

14 Ferri M, Amato L, Davoli M. Alcoholics Anonymous and other 12-step programmes for alcohol dependence. Cochrane Database Syst Rev. 2009; **19**(3): CD005032.

15 White W. *Slaying the Dragon: the history of addiction treatment and recovery in America.* Chicago, IL: Chestnut Health Systems/Lighthouse Institute; 1998.

16 Center for Substance Abuse Treatment. *Therapeutic Community Curriculum: trainer's manual.* DHHS Publication No. (SMA) 06–4121. Rockville, MD: Substance Abuse and Mental Health Services Administration; 2006.

17 National Institute on Drug Abuse (NIDA). *Research Report Series: therapeutic communities.* Bethesda, MD: US Department of Health and Human Sciences and National Institute of Health; 2002.

18 Jainchill N, Hawke J, DeLoen G, *et al.* Adolescent in therapeutic communities: one-year post-treatment outcomes. *J Psychoactive Drugs.* 2000; **32**(1): 81–94. Cited in Center for Substance Abuse Treatment (CSAT). *Treatment of Adolescents with Substance Abuse Disorders.* Treatment Improvement Protocol (TIP) Series, no 32. Rockville, MD: Substance Abuse and Mental Health Services Administration (US); 1999.

19 Petry NM. *Contingency Management for Substance Abuse Treatment: a guide to implementing this evidenced-based practice.* New York, NY: Routledge; 2011.

20 Stanger C, Budney AJ. Contingency management approaches for adolescent substance use disorders. *Child Adolesc Psychiatr Clin N Am.* 2010; **19**(3): 547–62.

21 Stanger C, Budney AJ, Kamon JL, *et al.* A randomized trial of contingency management for adolescent marijuana abuse and dependence. *Drug Alcohol Depend.* 2009; **105**(3): 240–7.

22 National Treatment Agency (NTA). *Guidance for the Pharmacological Management of Substance Misuse among Young People.* London: National Treatment Agency for Substance Misuse; 2009.

23 Sullivan JT, Sykora K, Schneiderman J, *et al.* Assessment of alcohol withdrawal: the revised Clinical Institute Withdrawal Assessment for Alcohol scale (CIWA – Ar). *Br J Addict.* 1989; **84**: 1353–7.

24 National Institute of Clinical Excellence (NICE). *Drug Misuse: opioid detoxification.* London: National Institute for Health and Clinical Excellence; 2007. www.nice.org. uk/nicemedia/live/11813/35999/35999.pdf

25 Lingford-Hughes AR, Welch S, Peters L, *et al.* Evidence-based guidelines for the pharmacological management of substance abuse, harmful use, addiction and comorbidity: recommendations from BAP. *J Psychopharmacology.* 2012; **26**(7): 899–952.

26 Budney AJ, Hughes JR. The cannabis withdrawal syndrome. *Curr Opin Psychiatry.* 2006; **19**(3): 233–8.

27 Schierenbeck T, Riemann D, Berger M, *et al.* Effect of illicit recreational drugs upon sleep: cocaine, Ecstasy and marijuana. *Sleep Med Rev.* 2008; **12**(5): 381–9.

28 Smyth BP, Kernan K, Fagan J. Outcome of heroin dependent adolescents commenced on opiate substitution treatment. *J Subst Abuse Treat.* 2012; **42**(1): 35–44.

29 Dolan K, Rouen D, Kimber J. An overview of the use of urine, hair, sweat and saliva to detect drug use. *Drug Alcohol Rev.* 2004; **23**(2): 213–17.

30 Irwin CE. To test or not to test: screening for substance use in adolescents. *J Adolesc Health.* 2006; **38**(4): 329–31.

31 Roche AM, Pidd K, Bywood P, *et al. Drug Testing in Schools: evidence, impacts and alternatives.* Canberra: Australian National Council on Drugs; 2008.

CHAPTER 12

Developing substance use policies

INTRODUCTION

Disruptive behaviour, late attendance, lack of engagement, poor performance, truancy, falling asleep in class, poor or absent homework and substance-affected behaviour are some of the problems that substance use can bring to school or youth-working communities. Some of these problems may have other causes, such as staying awake until the early hours of the morning gaming or on social networks. However, they can be rooted in substance use.

The European Schools Survey Project on Alcohol and Other Drugs is a study carried out every 4 years with 15- to 16-year-olds in mainstream schools. Thirty-six countries now participate in this study. In 2011, 13% of students reported using cannabis in the last year, with 7% using in the last 30 days.[1] Every school and youth group can expect to encounter individuals who are involved in substance use at some stage. How should one respond to a teenager who has been found using or in possession of drugs or alcohol? Should the teenager be removed or given a reprimand? Should the incident result in a conversation that provides information or advice? Should parents or police be involved?

Ideally every school or youth group should have a substance use policy. The development and implementation of this policy will help in responding to these issues. As with all policy development, they should not be seen as an end product; instead, they require intermittent reviewing to ensure best practice. This chapter will give an overview of the impact of substance use in schools and youth groups, which will set the context for looking at substance misuse policy development. We will explore what a policy is, why one is needed and what should be included.

IMPACT OF SUBSTANCE MISUSE IN SCHOOLS AND YOUTH GROUPS

The use of substances by adolescents can have a significant impact on those around them. Naturally we all think of the effect on the individual, family and friends, but classmates, members of the school community and youth clubs are also likely to be affected. Substance use can bring with it decreased participation and poor work ethos resulting in lower grades.[2] Youth workers and teachers can become disheartened, as despite their best efforts, they may feel they are working against the tide. Young people may leave or avoid the group. Having to respond to the problems created by substance use presents a distraction from the core mission of an organisation. A service will have concerns about the teenager but will also have legitimate concerns about potential reputational damage if they are not seen to deal with the problem appropriately. Likewise, the organisation has to protect other adolescents attending their service and so may be worried about the possible negative effects of having someone who is using drugs remain a member.

Drug supply and selling are common problems associated with drug use. Often what starts as getting cannabis for a friend gradually develops into a situation where a teen can create a free supply for him- or herself. In time the teen may earn cash directly. While most adolescents would not see themselves as a 'drug dealer', the role of the contact person can evolve into that role. This brings with it concerning risks. Debts, threats and violence are possible by-products of the activity of procuring and selling illicit drugs. A school or youth group can find that they have to deal with these events, even though they involve only a small percentage of young people. Substance use policies need to cover these behaviours and events alongside providing education, monitoring and response in relation to substance use.

WHAT IS A POLICY?

A policy is an agreed statement of intention that clearly sets out an organisation's views with respect to a particular matter. It is a set of principles that provide direction. A policy will clarify what approach will be taken in response to particular dilemmas. If the policy content has legal implications, these will be enshrined in the document.

Schools create policies in line with their national department of education guidelines. National policies provide the overall influence for policy development within a country or state. Different countries have different approaches to dealing with substance use problems. The aim of the National Drug Control Strategy in the United States is to reduce the use of drugs, whereas the goal of Australian policy is to reduce the harm caused by drugs.[3] The United States has laws about alcohol use that are stricter than Australia or most European countries. The United States takes a 'zero tolerance' approach to drug use, whereas Australia and most European countries take a harm reduction approach. These differing approaches are driven by and reflected in policy development.

A harm reduction policy is an approach to substance misuse that attempts to reduce the harm that occurs, and acknowledging that while the abuse of drugs is harmful to both the individual and the community, complete prohibition of drug use is an unattainable goal.[4] Research evidence indicates that harm reduction policies provide many benefits to adults; however, the blanket approach used with adults cannot be applied to teens. Harm reduction interventions need to be specifically tailored to the developmental stage of an individual and take their social context into consideration.[4]

Developmental stages are not fixed events in childhood but are, instead, broad guidelines. Adolescence is the developmental period between childhood and early adulthood, beginning at approximately 10–12 years and ending at 18–22 years.[5] Because of the unique pace of development of each teen, and each teen's differing social contexts, care is needed when sharing harm reduction information. Harm reduction strategies suggest that safe use of drugs should be advocated where drug use is happening – for example, encouraging the use of glass rather than plastic bongs for smoking cannabis. However, a practitioner has a responsibility to ensure that the adolescent does not construe this as approval of the use. There is a seemingly contradictory task for the practitioner: to let the adolescent know that it is best for his or her physical, emotional and mental health that he or she does not smoke cannabis, while also communicating information that helps the adolescent to use safely if he or she decides to. Research indicates that holding clear alcohol-specific rules to delay drinking has a protective effect.[6] One can extrapolate that the same probably applies to cannabis. The contradiction stands that a practitioner is trying to motivate a minor to not use substances and also motivate the minor to use safely. The importance of the former must not be lost when working with adolescents with a harm reduction approach.

Harm reduction policy proponents sometimes push for legalisation, or certainly decriminalisation, of certain drugs. There is ongoing debate between policymakers, legislators, lobbyists and service providers. It is suggested that their illegality serves only to criminalise users and is not a useful harm reduction measure.[7] While there is no desire to criminalise adolescents, there is a risk that lax application of the law in relation to cannabis use does not support the young cannabis user to make changes that will benefit him or her. Rather, it gives a message that cannabis use it not a big deal.

Societal attitudes to adolescents' use of alcohol in some countries is mixed, with many choosing not to adhere to existing legislation and giving a spurious rationale for their failure, such as difficulty knowing the exact age of a teenager.

While adolescents are encouraged to make wise choices that will benefit their development, they are often failed repeatedly by poor governance that does not challenge lax application of licensing laws. It is difficult to imagine how governance of the sale of other mood-altering substances, if they were legalised, would be any different, thus putting young people at further risk.

Reflective practice

- What policy approach do you or your organisation embrace?
- What are the advantages and disadvantages of this position?

WHY HAVE POLICIES?

Policies communicate the philosophy of an organisation to those within it and to the general public. They provide a sense of how an organisation works and its position on a variety of topics. The boundaries for the smooth running of organisational life are laid out. This removes the necessity of revisiting similar issues each time they arise.

A well-developed policy will be devised by the entire organisation, or at least by representatives at every level. This allows for full ownership of the decisions made in the process. An inclusive approach promotes greater understanding of policies – what they contain and how they are applied. In the school context, this means involving students, teachers, parents and other staff members so that the policy reflects the views of all, or at least of the majority.[8] Most schools have developed and implemented substance use policies and have drug education and prevention initiatives imbedded in curricula. Youth organisations also have similar policies at local and national level. Organisations' national policies can be taken by any youth worker or group of adolescents and used as discussion points to formulate the local application of the national policy. It is beneficial to those delivering and participating in youth groups that they are encouraged to take ownership of policies. This local application allows for cultural nuances to be included. The ethic of the organisation can then become meaningful to the adolescents it hopes to guide. Community application of policies also allows the possibility of feedback for the organisation, so that it is operating in a manner that is relevant to the local context.

An organisation may adopt either a harm reduction or a prohibitionist stance, or it may try to maintain the balance between both. Its goal may be to prevent the use of substances and/or to encourage those who are already using to stop or reduce drug use. Policies that deal with substance misuse are among those that have been seen to be least effective. This should prompt us to continue to be rigorous in our efforts to find ways to support adolescents in making healthy decisions around their use of substances.

Harm reduction dilemma

- What is your personal position in relation to substance use policies for teenagers – harm reduction or abstinence?
- What are the potential negative impacts of providing harm reduction information to a mixed-age group of teenagers?
- How does your position fit with your country's child protection guidelines and legislation?

WHAT NEEDS TO BE INCLUDED IN A SUBSTANCE MISUSE POLICY?

While schools and youth groups have common features, each one will have particular issues related to substance use that require an individually tailored policy. Careful consideration must be given to identify the difficulties that affect an organisation and to address them.

However, it is important to clarify that the policy applies to all behaviour and practice related to substance use. A policy should include guidelines for staff as well as students' substance use. For instance, what will the organisational response be if students report that a teacher comes to class intoxicated or hungover? All activities prohibited by the substance misuse policy should be outlined clearly and precisely. The policy may need to have specific sections dealing with use of tobacco, alcohol, volatiles and illicit drugs.

Substance misuse policies should cover the following topics.

- *Health promotion*: the policy will describe the content and delivery of the health promotion programme addressing substance misuse issues. Aims of drug education can include increasing staff and youth knowledge of drug use and related issues. In addition, a programme may seek to present a variety of opinions and attitudes towards drug use and support analysis and critique of these. This approach facilitates open discussion and promotes trust and confidence building, which increases the likelihood of help-seeking if needed. Knowledge of up-to-date information on sources of help should be provided.
- *Confidentiality*: the substance misuse policy must be congruent with other policies in the organisation. All policies should be cross-referenced with one another. Confidentiality boundaries in relation to substance misuse must comply with ethical and legal requirements regarding adolescents.
- *Staff training*: many staff members may not feel comfortable dealing with

substance use issues, for a variety of reasons. Therefore, there may be a need for high-quality training.

- *Management of drugs and medicines within school boundaries and on school trips*: substance misuse policy should detail the who, what, where, when and how of looking after medication for staff, students and youth group members.

- *Management of incidents related to substance misuse*: staff are best placed to decide the most appropriate response to tackling substance use within their school or group. If a pupil is suspected of being under the influence of substances, the school must prioritise the safety of the teenager and those around them. Medical intervention should be provided if necessary. Referral to counselling or pastoral resources should be considered, and to a specialist service if needed. If there is uncertainty about what is needed, an assessment at a specialist service may help. A teenager may disclose that they or members of their family are missing substances or they may be found in possession of a substance. All eventualities should be covered by the policy. A balance of a pastoral approach with a discipline response is best. Balance the needs of the individual pupils concerned with those of the wider community. There is debate about drug testing in schools (*see* Chapter 11 for more information) and the policy should outline the approach to be taken. Ideally, local substance use treatment services should be identified in the policy.

- *Partnership with parents*: best practice indicates that parents should be included in the development of substance use policies. Parents offer other perspectives and possibly provide local knowledge and information. Inviting parents to participate also presents a more congruent message to youth.

- *Consequences for breaches of policy guidelines*: UK Department of Education guidelines suggest that 'exclusion should not be the automatic response to a drug incident and permanent exclusion should only be used in serious cases'.[8] The consequences of breaching the policy should be clearly stated, such as a 'three strikes and you're out' approach to expulsion. However, it may be more useful to describe a hierarchy of consequences or incentives. For instance, if a student blatantly uses illicit substances in a school or club, an automatic dismissal might be appropriate, whereas lesser offences could warrant a less extreme penalty. Suspensions are often used as consequences. It is important to bear in mind that a teenager who displays challenging behaviours may not be disturbed by being excluded from school and so they do not experience the response as a deterrent. In fact they may see it as a reward! Depending on the circumstances, parents or the police may need to be contacted.

- *Implementation of the policy*: a policy should be publicised within the organisation and made available to parents, students or youth group participants. A locally adapted version can be made available for youth group members.
- *Review and update*: a review date should be included and a senior staff member nominated to take responsibility for updating the policy.

BEST PRACTICE IN DEVELOPING SUBSTANCE USE POLICIES

A whole-school approach is best practice in relation to health promotion in schools; development of school substance misuse policies should be treated the same way. In youth groups, the same ethos is helpful in adapting organisational policies at local level. This fosters reflection on the issues and promotes ownership of all decisions. This process is as important as the policy itself.

This can be achieved by taking the steps outlined in Box 12.1 which are considered best practice for schools. They are equally applicable to youth groups, as they facilitate the policy becoming a live document. By live document we mean a real document that is referred to regularly for guidance and, importantly, edited to reflect actual practice.

BOX 12.1 Guidelines for developing a substance use policy for schools[9]

- Step 1: Establish a core committee to develop the policy
- Step 2: Study relevant resource documents and legislation
- Step 3: Review the current situation regarding substance use policy issues
- Step 4: Prepare a draft policy statement
- Step 5: Publicise, revise, amend and finalise the draft policy
- Step 6: Ratify, circulate and implement the agreed policy
- Step 7: Monitor, review and evaluate the policy

Step 1: Establish a core committee to develop the policy

In schools the committee should include students, parents, teachers, ancillary staff and those working in related organisations. In youth groups the group coordinator, any youth leader and representatives from a youth committee can form a subcommittee to develop local policy. Equally, organisational or government policy can be applied at local level. This inclusive approach not only supports the process of policy development but also sets a foundation that supports adolescents who experience problematic substance use.

Step 2: Study relevant resource documents and legislation

This task can be shared and can provide useful learning for all involved. Summaries and key points of relevant documents can be used to make this task manageable. Resource documents can include policy recommendations from the Department of Education, national youth organisations or national drug websites.

Step 3: Review the current situation regarding substance use policy issues

Having a mix of participants on a committee will give a broader response when issues related to substance use are discussed. Reviewing the current situation could mean carrying out a small research survey among the student group about their attitudes and experience of substance use. Another approach to gathering opinion and involving others is to organise a World Café group to discuss the topic with representatives from various classes or youth groups. World Café is a format for hosting group dialogue (*see* Box 12.2). It can be modified to meet a variety of needs.

Step 4: Prepare a draft policy statement

It is often unhelpful to take an existing policy and craft it to suit your own organisation. The document can be less meaningful and relevant than if the headings described in Box 12.1 are taken and the issues fleshed out for the specific environment.

Step 5: Publicise, revise, amend and finalise the draft policy

Circulate your draft policy and seek feedback on it. Ensure the board or management committee endorses the policy.

Step 6: Ratify, circulate and implement the agreed policy

The policy is communicated to all the relevant people and, if necessary, a date is set for an information session, to ensure all staff have the knowledge and skills to implement it. Set a date to review the policy.

Step 7: Monitor, review and evaluate the policy

Examine the school's practice, comparing and contrasting it with the school's policy. Failure to review the policy can result in staff moving away from decisions and actions that they had agreed upon. Situations can change over time and the local environment or local drug culture may demand a new approach.

BOX 12.2 World Café

1 Setting

Create a 'special' environment, most often modelled after a café (i.e. three to seven small round tables, with four chairs at each). You can use an optional 'talking stick' item. Each table has flip chart paper with several prompt questions related to the topic under discussion (i.e. What does our school community think about drug and alcohol misuse?).

2 Welcome and introduction

The host begins by welcoming participants and introducing the World Café process.

3 Small group rounds

The process begins with the first of three or more rounds of conversation for the small groups seated around a table. A host at each table takes notes on a flip chart. At the end of 5–10 minutes, each member of the group moves to a different, new table. This movement creates a cross-fertilisation of ideas. The host remains at the table for the next round, welcomes the next group and briefly fills them in on conversations in the previous round.

4 Questions

Each round is prefaced with questions to prompt conversation about substance issues in the school or club community, and possible responses. The same questions can be used for more than one round, or previous contributions can prompt the next conversation.

5 Harvest

After the small groups, individuals are invited to share insights from their conversations with the large group. These ideas are also gathered. The basic process is simple yet generative. The content of all the flip charts will provide rich information.

Note: see www.theworldcafe.com/publications.html

CONCLUSION

Is your policy a living document that serves the whole community or is it simply paperwork that exists to comply with a requirement that it is seen to exist? Does it reflect what actually happens in your organisation? Inclusive policy development can be an intervention in itself to respond to substance use within schools or clubs. The policy lays out a clear description of what will and what won't be accepted and how difficulties are responded to. A clear substance misuse policy ensures that when problems arise they are dealt with in a transparent and measured way. It is vital that the policy is reviewed regularly to ensure that it reflects actual practice.

KEY POINTS

- Policies offer information and guidance when dealing with drug and alcohol issues.
- Adolescents need the clarity and support of clear and effective drug and alcohol policies.
- A whole organisation approach to policy development creates an environment where the process is as productive as the end result.
- A living policy document is most supportive of the community that it serves.

REFERENCES

1 Hibell B, Guttormsson U, Ahlström S, *et al. The 2011 ESPAD Report: substance use among students in 36 European Countries.* Stockholm: Swedish Council for Information on Alcohol and Other Drugs (CAN); 2012.

2 Haase T, Pratschke J. *Risk and Protection Factors for Substance Use Among Young People: a comparative study of early school-leavers and school-attending students.* Dublin: The Stationery Office; 2010.

3 Beyers JM, Evans-Whipp T, Mathers M, *et al.* A cross-national comparison of school drug policies in Washington State, United States, and Victoria, Australia. *J Sch Health.* 2005; **75**(4): 134–140.

4 Bonomo YA, Bowes G. Putting harm reduction into an adolescent context. *J Paediatr Child Health.* 2001; **37**(1): 5–8.

5 Santrock JW. *Child Development.* 7th ed. Madison, WI: Brown & Benchmark; 1996.

6 Mares SH, Lichtwarck-Aschoff A, Burk WJ, *et al.* Parental alcohol-specific rules and alcohol use from early adolescence to young adulthood. *J Child Psychol Psychiatry.* 2012; **53**(7): 798–805.

7 Ryall G, Butler S. The great Irish head shop controversy. *Drug-Educ Prev Polic.* 2011; **18**(4): 303–11.

8 Department for Education; Association of Chief Police Officers. *DfE and ACPO Drug Advice for Schools.* London: Department for Education; 2012. Available at: www.gov. uk/government/uploads/system/uploads/attachment_data/file/209993/DfE_and_ACPO_drug_advice_for_schools.pdf (accessed 10 August 2013).

9 Department for Education. *Guideline for Developing a School Substance Use Policy.* Dublin: Department for Education; 2002. Available at: www.education.i.e./en/ Schools-Colleges/Information/Post-Primary-School-Policies/si_substance_use.pdf (accessed 5 January 2013).

CHAPTER 13

Substance use and mental health

INTRODUCTION

Many people working with adolescent substance users have concerns about mental health and psychological problems. This is understandable given that almost all studies examining mental illness among adolescent substance users find that they have substantially increased rates of mental health problems compared with adolescents who don't use drugs.

MENTAL ILLNESS VERSUS PSYCHOLOGICAL PROBLEMS

Most people have a clear idea of what a psychological problem is. When we discuss psychological problems we think of depression or mood problems, poor self-esteem, anger or suicide. Despite a general familiarity with the term 'psychological problem', there is no agreed definition. Mental illness, on the other hand, is more complicated and debated. Mental illnesses are clearly defined disorders or syndromes that are diagnosed and treated by mental health services. Psychiatry is the branch of medicine that is concerned with the identification and treatment of mental illness. So all psychiatrists are medical doctors and psychiatry has become synonymous with medications for the treatment of mental illness. However, in reality, the treatment of mental illness requires a large array of medical, psychological and social interventions, generally delivered by a multidisciplinary team.

When it comes to mental illnesses, there are two classification systems: the International Classification of Diseases, known as the ICD-10, and the Diagnostic and Statistical Manual of Mental Disorders (DSM), known as DSM-IV-TR. As a general rule, European countries use the ICD. These diagnostic guidelines seek to ensure that diagnoses are made in a consistent manner by psychiatrists across the world. Their task is to distinguish symptoms or problems from illnesses or disorders. Everyone feels sad or low in mood at times, but fewer people have a depressive *illness*. The diagnostic guidelines seek to define where the line is between 'ordinary' sadness and a depressive illness. Use of these guidelines to diagnose substance dependence was discussed in Chapter 7.

A point of confusion for those who don't come from a psychiatry perspective is the fact that many people who present with psychological problems (e.g. self-harming) may not meet the criteria for a mental illness using DSM or ICD. As a result, when they present to mental health services they may not be offered a service. This can lead to significant annoyance for the individual, his or her friends and family, and professionals from other agencies that are trying to help the individual. Importantly, while substance use disorders are defined by the ICD and DSM systems, they are generally not seen as mental illnesses. As such, treatment for them is usually the responsibility of substance use services that are separate from the mental health services. However, doctors specialising in addiction are increasingly arguing that substance dependence is a mental or brain disorder.

DUAL DIAGNOSIS

Dual diagnosis (DD) is a term used to describe a situation where a substance use disorder and a mental illness occur at the same time. Other terms such as co-occurring or co-morbid disorders are also used. As there are many substances that can be used, as well as a wide range of mental illnesses, there is a never-ending list of possible combinations. For example, alcohol misuse may co-occur with depression or an eating disorder. Likewise, schizophrenia may co-occur with alcohol, or cannabis misuse. What we do know is that DD is very common, with 50%–90% of adolescents with a substance use disorder also having a mental illness.[1,2] The figures vary from study to study but it can be accepted that when working with adolescents with substance use problems it is more likely that they have a mental health problem than not.

Accepting that many of these adolescents have a co-occurring mental illness often leads to the chicken-and-egg debate. The reality is that this is a needless and academic debate because, first, it is often unanswerable and leads only to educated guesses and, second, it frequently makes little difference to treatment. Broadly speaking, there are five ways for DD to present itself.

1 Substance use *causes* mental illness: in some cases the use of a substance can bring about a mental illness, or at least symptoms that mirror a mental illness. For example, a drug-induced psychosis.

2 Mental illness *causes* substance use: having a mental illness can lead to someone using a substance as a way of coping. For example, smoking cannabis to reduce anxiety.

3 The mental illness may not cause but it does *exacerbate* the coexisting

substance use disorder, or vice versa. For example, while a person is depressed, they may be poorly motivated to address their cannabis use disorder. If a person with schizophrenia abuses amphetamines, this may result in an escalation of their psychotic symptoms.

4 The *treatment* of one condition may cause the other. For example, a person with an anxiety disorder who is prescribed diazepam may misuse this medication and become dependent upon it.

5 Mental illness and substance use co-occur but are *unrelated*. Here the individual has two disorders, but this may be no more than an unfortunate coincidence.

When you meet an adolescent, it is not always possible to know which of these situations applies. Take, for example, an adolescent who presents with psychotic symptoms and smokes cannabis. It is known that psychosis and cannabis are related – those who smoke cannabis are more likely to experience psychotic symptoms.[3,4] There is a tendency for many professionals to assume that any adolescent who presents with cannabis use and psychosis has a drug-induced psychosis. The reality is that most people who are psychotic have not used cannabis and most people who use cannabis are not psychotic. We cannot know whether a particular client would have become psychotic or not if they had not smoked cannabis. Hence it is impossible to determine the relationship between the drug use and the mental health problem.

Naturally, if the person stops using the substance we often see a change in his or her mental health symptoms, which would indicate a relationship between the two, but it is not always possible to get someone to stop. So the cannabis user might continue to smoke despite being advised that this is likely to make his psychotic symptoms worse. In some instances, we have come across situations where mental health services refuse to treat someone because they continue to use a substance. This seems patently unfair. We do not refuse to treat someone's high blood pressure because they have not lost weight. Nor do we refuse to treat someone's diabetes because they continue to eat biscuits. Unfortunately, poor adherence with treatment and healthy lifestyle advice is extremely common across the full spectrum of healthcare problems.

Substance abuse services will often avoid working with someone with a mental illness. They may decide that a patient's mental health needs are beyond their competence. This is most likely to occur where adolescents present with co-occurring psychotic symptoms or suicidal behaviours. Unfortunately, this can result in scenarios where adolescents with complex needs are denied treatment by both mental health and substance abuse treatment services. Ideally, both problems need to be treated together, with the two services working collaboratively.

OVERVIEW OF SUBSTANCE USE AND VARIOUS MENTAL ILLNESSES

The diagnoses that are applied can vary slightly from DSM to ICD. However when thinking of psychiatric diagnoses it is worth remembering that, in general, they:

- each have a specific set of symptoms and the person must have a minimum number of these to fit the criteria
- these symptoms must affect functioning in some way such as socially, academically or in relationships.

Affective/mood disorders

Depression and mania are the two main types of mood disorders. Depression is characterised by a persistently low mood. By persistent we mean that the low mood is evident most days and lasts most of the day. For example, someone who has low mood when in school but is fine the rest of the time is unlikely to meet this criterion. In addition, this low mood must be different from how the person normally presents. Depression is the most common co-occurring psychiatric disorder among adolescents, with rates of 24%–35% reported in research. In practice, many clients with substance use problems have difficulties related to mood even if they do not meet the criteria for depressive disorder. It is not hard to see why the effects of drug use, such as declining performance in school or sports, disrupted relationships and drug debts, would lead to lower mood. Likewise many people who have depression find that taking a substance makes them feel better, temporarily at least. It is unlikely that this will prove to be a long-term solution and often it reinforces the problems they were down about in the first place.

Mania is where the person experiences a euphoric episode often characterised by increased energy and confidence and a decreased need for sleep. Manic episodes are a feature of bipolar affective disorder (BPAD), which is sometimes called 'manic depression'. This can lead to significant problems as the person becomes impulsive and engages in risky behaviour. Many of the stimulant drugs give an effect similar to a manic episode, but these resolve quickly once the drug wears off. In reality, few adolescents present to substance abuse services with manic episodes. For example, an American study[5] reported only 3.3% of clients had BPAD and a study of 144 teenagers attending our service did not identify any clients with BPAD.[6]

Psychosis

Psychosis is a complicated concept for the simple reason that it is very broad. However, here we will confine it to discussing psychiatric problems that manifest themselves with three main symptoms.

1 *Delusions*: these are persistently held false beliefs. Many people using

drugs, particularly cannabis, report feeling paranoid. Typically this is no more than a type of social anxiety symptom arising from heightened self-consciousness. For example, a person may think that laughter in a room following their arrival is due to them, and they may leave. However, they can accept that the people may not have been laughing at them. This is not a paranoid delusion. If the person stated that the other people in the room could hear their thoughts, then this bizarre belief would indicate a delusion. In other cases, the beliefs can be extremely odd, such as thinking you are able to fly and so forth. Naturally, these beliefs can lead to people doing very dangerous things, including attempting to fly by jumping from heights.

2 *Hallucinations*: these refer to situations where people experience something through one of their senses that is not actually there. In other words, it is created by their mind but experienced as real. Most commonly, people hear a voice, i.e. an auditory hallucination. However, there are four other senses so we can have hallucinations that are visual, tactile (touch), olfactory (smell) or gustatory (taste). Most commonly, in schizophrenia, people hear voices. Nevertheless, fleeting auditory hallucinations often happen with drugs such as cannabis. Visual hallucinations are mainly associated with drugs such as LSD or magic mushrooms. Hallucinations of smell, touch and taste are less commonly due to drug use and, when they occur, are often associated with withdrawal rather than intoxication.

3 *Thought disorder*: the individual has difficulty organising their thoughts and this presents as a disorganised pattern in speech such as not finishing sentences or shifting from topic to topic. This makes the conversation hard to follow for the listener.

Importantly, people who experience delusions or hallucinations can engage in productive, meaningful conversations. They are not stupid or confused. They may believe that a television newscaster is deliberately mocking them. They may intermittently hear a voice that tells them they are evil. However, they may still be able to engage in an informed, articulate conversation about the weather, the political situation or their substance use. Consequently, as long as they are not completely preoccupied by their delusions or hallucinations, they can participate in treatment for the substance use problems. There are a number of types of psychosis including schizophrenia, drug-induced psychosis and mania. In reality, most adolescent services do not see many teenagers with psychotic symptoms – Wise, *et al.*[5] did not report any psychosis other than those with mania, and our study reported rates of psychosis of only 5%.[6] However, because of links between cannabis and psychosis it is one mental illness that is often talked about – parents will often say to us that they are worried that their child will get schizophrenia. The reality is that most people who get psychotic never used drugs and most people who use drugs never get psychotic. However, they are at an increased risk of becoming psychotic, so it is worth keeping it in mind.

Attention deficit hyperactivity disorder

Attention deficit hyperactivity disorder (ADHD) is one of the common childhood mental health problems. It is sometimes known as attention deficit disorder but they are the same thing, and ADHD is the proper term. About 6%–12% of children are affected by it throughout the world.[7] Wise, *et al.*[5] found 11% of their sample had ADHD, while in our study almost 21% had ADHD.[6] ADHD is a disorder characterised by three main symptoms: (1) hyperactivity, (2) poor concentration and (3) impulsivity. You don't need to be a psychiatrist to see that these symptoms might make someone more likely to try drugs, either to manage how he or she feels or because he or she makes poorer choices because of the impulsivity. It is worth noting that ADHD must have its onset before the age of 7 and so it would be unlikely that the substance use would commence before this. Sometimes the ADHD is not diagnosed until after drug use commences, which complicates things.

What is clear is that children with untreated ADHD are at greater risk of developing substance use disorders as adolescents. Psychiatrists are sometimes reluctant to prescribe medications to those who have ADHD and are abusing substances because some ADHD medications have the potential to be abused. The reality is that those who do not have their ADHD treated are at most risk of substance use and so it is vital that adolescents who have ADHD receive appropriate care. In cases where clients with ADHD commence substance use, this should be treated in conjunction with the ADHD while being vigilant to ensure medications are not misused.[8] Simply stopping the ADHD medications is unlikely to bring about positive results.

Conduct disorder and oppositional defiant disorder

Conduct disorder (CD) and oppositional defiant disorder (ODD) are two disorders that are commonly discussed in child and adolescent mental health services. ODD is a persistent pattern of defiance and disobedience towards authority figures, whereas CD is a persistent pattern of breaking societal norms and violating the rights of others.[9] About 3% of children meet criteria for ODD, with a further 7% of girls and 12% of boys meeting criteria for CD.[10] CD is associated with more antisocial and aggressive behaviour than ODD and, officially, ODD cannot be diagnosed in someone who meets criteria for CD. Therefore, someone should only have a diagnosis of either CD or ODD, although we have come across situations where individuals are diagnosed with both. It is not surprising that CD and ODD are common among those who misuse substances, with about one in four young people attending substance abuse treatment meeting criteria.[5] Compare the two case studies in Box 13.1 – while both Tom and Adam have the same level of substance use their histories are different.

BOX 13.1 Case studies of conduct disorder

Tom

Tom is a 16-year-old boy. He has been smoking cannabis for 2 years and daily for about 6 months. He has never been in trouble with the police and his parents are surprised by his drug use. Previously, he got on well in school and had many hobbies. However, he has got into trouble in school recently for skipping classes and not having his homework done. He has also stopped playing basketball, which he was passionate about.

Adam

Adam is a 16-year-old boy. He has been smoking cannabis for about 2 years and daily for about 6 months. His parents are frustrated as they feel he is always in trouble. Throughout primary school, teachers complained about his angry, difficult behaviour. He rarely adhered to rules at home. He has been suspended from school numerous times for skipping classes, fighting with fellow pupils and arguing with teachers. He was also arrested by the police for vandalism and fighting.

ODD is more commonly diagnosed in pre-teens, with many of these eventually going on to meet criteria for the more serious CD. Those who have a later onset of CD have a more favourable outcome than those who develop it earlier in life.[11] With both ODD or CD, there are a few points that are important to bear in mind.

- They make adolescents more likely to misuse substances.
- They can coexist with other mental health problems, particularly ADHD, so a full assessment of mental health is advisable.
- They are treatable and should not simply be dismissed as bold behaviour.
- Most of the research suggests that interventions with parents (such as Functional Family Therapy – *see* Chapter 8) are particularly valuable with both ODD[12] and CD.[11]

Anxiety disorders

Anxiety disorder is a term used to describe a range of psychiatric disorders where the key feature is intense anxiety or fear. Some of the more common anxiety disorders are outlined here.

- *Post-traumatic stress disorder*: where the individual experiences nightmares, flashbacks, sustained anxiety and hyper-vigilance following a traumatic event such as an assault.
- *Social anxiety*: where the individual experiences intense fear of and usually avoids situations where they believe they are likely to be exposed to criticism by others. For example they may avoid talking to members of the opposite sex.
- *Obsessive–compulsive disorder*: here the person experiences recurrent thoughts (obsessions) which cause them distress or anxiety. For example, they may think that door handles are covered in germs. As a result, they have an urge to repeat a behaviour (i.e. a compulsion) that will reduce their distress, such as hand washing.
- *Panic disorder*: when the person experiences intense anxiety attacks and feel they are going to die. As a result they avoid situations where panic may occur.
- *Phobias*: ongoing fears of specific situations or things. Common phobias include agoraphobia where the person is afraid of being in a situation where they may not be able to leave easily. Likewise, people may be afraid of specific things such as spiders. The key thing about phobias is that the person recognises that his or her level of anxiety is out of proportion to the actual danger, although this may not be true in young children.
- *Generalised anxiety disorder*: the name given to a situation where an individual experiences ongoing anxiety or worry that does not meet the other categories and often has features of many of them. It is of a persistent nature and is present most of the time.

Anxiety disorders cause the person significant impairment. For example, it interferes with his or her ability to go to school, socialise or take part in normal hobbies. There are conflicting reports in the literature about the relationship between anxiety and substance use, with some research suggesting that anxiety disorders may be a protective factor. This makes sense, as those with anxiety are *probably less likely to risk experimenting* with potentially harmful drugs. On the other hand, other studies suggest that those with anxiety disorders are more likely to abuse substances, which fits with a self-medicating theory. In other words, they feel anxious and use drugs to reduce the anxiety. In practice this can only be assessed on an individual basis and even then it can be hard to be sure. Rates of anxiety disorders among substance-abusing adolescents vary, but can be as high as 20%.[5] However, in our study only 6% of clients were diagnosed with an anxiety disorder.[6] When working with teenagers with substance use problems, it is important to explore if anxiety symptoms act as a trigger for their substance use. If so, they may be unlikely to cease use until they have been given alternative coping strategies to deal with these symptoms.

It is safe to assume that some adolescents may have anxiety symptoms brought on by substance use – the effects of many stimulants can present as similar to anxiety. Likewise many teenagers with anxiety problems may discover that substances help them to cope with the anxiety and so they are more likely to use again. This is not necessarily a sign of mental illness and is quite common. For example, many teenagers find it difficult to 'chat up' someone they fancy. They use substances, typically alcohol, as a way of giving them more confidence to enable them to do so. This is often referred to as 'Dutch courage'. This does not indicate an unhealthy level of anxiety on its own; rather, it indicates an unhealthy coping strategy.

Personality disorders

Personality disorders (PDs) are a form of disorder where the individual displays enduring patterns of perceiving, thinking, behaving and feeling that result in problems for the person across most aspects of his or her life. These patterns are stable and are established during adolescence or early adulthood. Notably, they tend to be persistent and cause considerable disruption to the individual's life. There are a variety of PDs depending on the particular presentation. One example of a common PD is borderline personality disorder, which is sometimes called emotionally unstable personality disorder. Individuals with borderline personality disorder experience frequent, but rapidly fluctuating, negative emotions. They are typically very insecure in relationships, think people are abandoning them and often engage in self-harm and other risky behaviours including unprotected sex and substance use.

BOX 13.2 A case study of a client with borderline personality disorder

Penny is a 17-year-old girl. She has a long history of contact with services. She was taken into care at various times in her childhood when her mother's drinking became particularly problematic. Penny reports being sexually abused by one of her mother's partners from age 9 to 11. Since the age of 13 she has smoked cannabis almost daily and since then she has sporadically used a variety of other drugs including alcohol, ecstasy, heroin and cocaine. She moves between the care system and staying with a variety of older boyfriends – most of whom are drug users. These relationships tend to be heated and intense and rarely last more than a few months. Penny herself admits she hates not having a boyfriend. She has inflicted cuts with razors to her arms on numerous occasions when she is upset but denies ever trying to kill herself.

There is often reluctance among clinicians to use the label PD when working with adolescents. One reason is the fact that the disorder tends to carry negative connotations as it comments on an individual's personality. Naturally, this can often be interpreted quite negatively. A more practical concern is that adolescence is frequently a difficult time during which personalities are evolving. It is therefore quite common for adolescents to present with quite striking and problematic personality characteristics during their teenage years, but these *don't always* persist into adulthood. Professionals do not want to land a diagnosis on someone, particularly one that is perceived as negative, when it may not last. In fact the ICD-10 criteria specifically state that the symptoms must start in childhood and persist into adulthood.[13] If someone *is* under 18 years of age, it can be argued that person cannot meet the criteria as the symptoms have yet to persist into adulthood.

The reality is that in many cases adolescents do present with features of the various PDs. A study published in 1993 that assessed the rates of PDs among 733 young people aged 9–21 years found rates of over 30% in the general population.[14] The general trend was for rates to peak at the start of the teenage years and decrease as children moved through adolescence and into adulthood with obsessive–compulsive, paranoid, narcissistic and borderline the most common subtypes. Bernstein and colleagues[14] also found that those who had a PD were more likely to have significant difficulties in a variety of areas including other psychiatric problems, trouble with police, poorer school and work performance and problems in interpersonal relationships. Findings like this have led to claims that professionals need to take PDs among adolescents seriously and intervene early so as to limit the problems they can cause.[15] Rather than standing back and hoping it doesn't persist into adulthood it is probably best to assume that they have a PD. Whether the actual diagnosis is officially made and shared with the teenager is a separate matter. If the teenager has a PD it is important that professionals bear this in mind. It might be quite useful for the substance use behaviour to be separated out from the behaviours associated with his or her PD. Progress could conceivably be made on both problems or only one.

Eating disorders

Eating disorders are one of the most commonly discussed teenage mental health problems. The two most common eating disorders are as follows.

1 *Anorexia nervosa* involves individuals self-restricting food intake to the point that they consistently maintain a weight that is too low for their height and age. By definition, malnutrition sets in and this can lead to physical health complications. There is often an overemphasis on the importance of body image and appearance and an overwhelming fear of gaining weight.

2 *Bulimia nervosa* is characterised by frequent binges of high-calorie food and, as a result, individuals resort to excessive exercising, vomiting or using medications such as laxatives to rid themselves of the calories they have taken in.

It is worth noting that bulimia, which affects about 2% of teens, is much more common than anorexia, and only about 5%–10% of those with an eating disorder are male.[16] It is unusual for teenagers with anorexia to abuse substances, unless they are doing so for the purposes of weight loss (e.g. amphetamines to suppress appetite). Substance use problems can certainly occur alongside bulimia. A large study in the United States of over 2000 dual diagnosed teenagers found that 5.5% of girls and 0.7% of boys had a diagnosis of an eating disorder.[17] Another study of 91 teenagers receiving inpatient treatment for substance abuse identified no eating disorders[5] and our study of 144 outpatients only identified one person with an eating disorder.[6]

Deliberate self-harm

Deliberate self-harm (DSH) is a term used to describe situations were individuals engage in a deliberate behaviour that results in harm to themselves, usually without the intention of killing themselves. DSH is not a mental illness itself but it is a sign of emotional distress and is associated with a variety of other mental health problems such as depression, personality and eating disorders. DSH can come in a variety of forms such as cutting, stabbing, burning or biting oneself. Less obvious forms can include picking at cuts, which prevents them from healing, banging your head against a wall or punching things.

DSH is surprisingly common among adolescents. A large study of over 30 000 14- to 17-year-olds from Australia, Belgium, England, Hungary, Ireland, the Netherlands and Norway found that 11.1% had self-harmed at least once.[18] In addition, rates of self-harm were over three times higher in girls than boys and the primary motivation tended to be to deal with pain or distress rather than a cry for help. In a Scottish study, worries about sexual orientation, history of sexual abuse, anxiety and self-esteem were all linked with repeat self-harm.[19] DSH among 14-year-olds has also been linked with poor relations with parents, a ruminative approach to dealing with problems, emotional, conduct, eating and attentional disorders as well as alcohol use.[20] Our study found that 27% of adolescents attending our service had self-harmed, with a significant gender imbalance – almost three out of five girls compared with one out of five boys.[6]

As previously noted, many drugs increase impulsivity and so the likelihood of self-harming may increase. When it comes to increasing impulsivity, alcohol and benzodiazepines are of particular concern. Also, self-harm is a predictor of actual completed suicide. This can generate major concern for adults who encounter adolescents with DSH. However, suicide occurs in only about 1 in every 10 000 adolescents, while DSH occurs in over 1 in 10. Therefore the ratio of adolescents who self-harm to those who complete suicide is about 1000 to 1. DSH deserves a proportionate response. It should not be dismissed, nor should it become the exclusive focus of attention unless it is associated with ongoing declared suicidal intent. In view of the association between substance use and suicidal behaviour, staff working with substance-using adolescents should obtain training in strategies to assess and manage these behaviours – for example, Applied Suicide Intervention Skills Training (see www.asist.org.uk/en/).

In many cases, DSH will present as one of the risky behaviours the teen presents with in addition to his or her substance use. Those working with the teen need to address both problems, but allow the adolescent to discuss his or her behaviour openly. This often requires a delicate balancing between taking appropriate steps to reduce risk and not alienating the client.

CONCLUSION

Substance use and mental health problems go hand in hand for many teenagers. It is hard to imagine how any professional who works with adolescents with substance use problems could avoid working with adolescents who also have mental health problems. This does not mean that every service has to be a DD service. Rather, it means that it is vital that they do not ignore the mental health needs of their substance-using clients and that they forge good inter-agency working with services who can help with the other needs. Just as a service for adolescent substance users might work closely with social work teams, they also need to work closely with mental health teams. The converse is also true – mental health services will also need to be able to address substance use within adolescents with mental health problems. In fact, the European Monitoring Centre for Drugs and Drug Addiction recently advised that children with psychiatric disorders should be viewed at particular risk of developing a substance use problem and should therefore be targeted for prevention programmes.[21] For more information on inter-agency working, please read Chapter 16. Unfortunately, mental health services excessively mystify substance use problems and substance use services mystify mental disorders. We argue that each service is strengthened by ensuring it employs some staff competent in the other area. Adolescent addiction services should include psychiatrists or psychiatric nurses, and adolescent mental health services should include staff skilled in substance use.

KEY POINTS

- Mental health problems are common among adolescent substance users.
- Mood problems, DSH, conduct disorder and ADHD are the most common mental health problems among adolescent substance users.
- Having both the substance use and mental health problems identified in a shorter time period is associated with better engagement with treatment.[17]
- Those working with adolescent substance users should actively seek to identify and deal with mental health problems and those who work with adolescents with mental health problems should actively seek to identify and deal with substance use problems.
- The basis of treatment is that substance abuse treatments still work for those who also have a mental health problem and mental health treatments also work for those who have a substance use disorder.[22]
- Motivational Interviewing has the most evidence for bringing about change in the short term and works, when combined with cognitive behavioural therapy, to bring about changes in mental state. Cognitive behavioural therapy alone (i.e. without Motivational Interviewing) is not well supported by research.[23]
- In order to ensure appropriate, proportionate responses to DSH and suicidal behaviour, staff in adolescent substance abuse services should obtain training in interventions such as Applied Suicide Intervention Skills Training.
- The argument about which came first is not so important – all the evidence suggests once identified, you just treat both the substance use and mental health problem concurrently.

FURTHER READING

- For an in-depth analysis of the area of DD, David Cooper produced a series of six books on the topic. For further information see http://46.175.49.77/Mental%20 Health%E2%80%93Substance%20Use/default.htm
- Kaminer Y, Bukstein OG, editors. *Adolescent Substance Abuse: psychiatric comorbidity and high-risk behaviours.* New York, NY: Routledge; 2008.

REFERENCES

1 Crome IB, Baldacchino A. The young person's perspective. In: Cooper DB, editor. *Responding in Mental Health: substance use.* London: Radcliffe; 2011. pp. 48–60.
2 James PD, Smyth BP. The child's perspective. In: Cooper DB, editor. *Responding in Mental Health: substance use.* London: Radcliffe; 2011. pp. 61–77.
3 Moore THM, Zammit S, Lingford-Hughes A, *et al.* Cannabis use and risk of psychotic

or affective mental health outcomes: a systematic review. *Lancet.* 2007; **370**(9584): 319–28.

4 Minozzi S, Davoli M, Bargagli AM, *et al.* An overview of systematic reviews on cannabis and psychosis: discussing apparently conflicting results. *Drug Alcohol Rev.* 2010; **29**(3): 304–17.

5 Wise BK, Cuffe SP, Fischer T. Dual diagnosis and successful participation of adolescents in substance abuse treatment. *J Subst Abuse Treat.* 2001; **21**(3): 161–5.

6 James PD, Smyth BP, Apantaku-Olajide T. Substance use and psychiatric disorders in Irish adolescents: a cross-sectional study of patients attending a substance abuse treatment service. *Ment Health Subst Abuse.* 2013; **6**(2): 124–32.

7 Biederman J, Favaone SV. Attention-deficit hyperactivity disorder. *Lancet.* 2005; **366**(9481): 237–48.

8 Edokpolo O, Nkire N, Smyth BP. Irish adolescents with ADHD and comorbid substance use disorder. *Ir J Psychol Med.* 2010; **27**(3): 148–51.

9 American Psychiatric Association. *Diagnostic and Statistical Manual of Mental Disorders.* 4th ed, text revision. Washington, DC: American Psychiatric Association; 2000.

10 Nock MK, Kazdin AE, Hiripi E, *et al.* Prevalence, subtypes, and correlates of DSM-IV conduct disorder in the National Comorbidity Survey Replication. *Psychol Med.* 2006; **36**(5): 699–710.

11 McGuiness TM. Update on conduct disorder. *J Psychosoc Nurs Ment Health Serv.* 2006; **44**(12): 21–5.

12 Hamilton SS, Armando J. Oppositional defiant disorder. *Am Fam Physician.* 2008; **78**(7): 861–6.

13 World Health Organization (WHO). *The ICD-10 Classification of Mental and Behavioural Disorders.* Geneva: WHO; 1992.

14 Bernstein DP, Cohen P, Velez CN, *et al.* Prevalence and stability of DSM-III-R personality disorders in a community-based survey of adolescents. *Am J Psychiatry.* 1993; **150**(8): 1237–43.

15 Bleiberg E. *Treating Personality Disorders in Children and Adolescents: a relational approach.* New York, NY: Guilford Press; 2001.

16 Herpertz S, Hagenah U, Vocks S, *et al.* The diagnosis and treatment of eating disorders. *Dtsch Arztebl Int.* 2011; **108**(40): 678–85.

17 Chi FW, Sterling S, Weisner C. Adolescents with co-occurring substance use and mental conditions in a private managed care health plan: prevalence, patient characteristics and treatment initiation and engagement. *Am J Addict.* 2006; **15**(Suppl 1): 67–79.

18 Scoliers G, Portzky G, Madge N, *et al.* Reasons for adolescent deliberate self-harm: a cry of pain and/or a cry for help? *Soc Psychiatry Psychiatr Epidemiol.* 2009; **44**(8): 601–7.

19 O'Connor RC, Rasmussen S, Hawton K. Predicting deliberate self-harm in adolescents: a six month prospective study. *Suicide Life Threat Behav.* 2009; **39**(4): 364–75.

20 Bjarehed J, Lundh LG. Deliberate self-harm in 14-year-old adolescents: how frequent is it, and how is it associated with psychopathology, relationship variables, and styles of emotional regulation? *Cogn Behav Ther.* 2008; **37**(1): 26–37.

21 EMCDDA. *Preventing Later Substance Use Disorders in At-Risk Children and Adolescents:*

a review of the theory and evidence base for indicated prevention. Luxembourg: Office for Official Publications of the European Communities; 2009. Available at: www.emcdda.europa.eu/publications/thematic-papers/indicated-prevention (accessed 11 August 2013).

22 Tiet QQ, Mausbach B. Treatments for patients with dual diagnosis: a review. *Alcohol Clin Exp Res.* 2007; **31**(4): 513–36.

23 Cleary M, Hunt GE, Matheson S, *et al.* Psychosocial treatments for people with co-occurring severe mental illness and substance misuse: systematic review. *J Adv Nurs.* 2009; **65**(2): 238–58.

CHAPTER 14

Substance use and sexual health

INTRODUCTION

Talking about sex sometimes tests the limits of a professional's comfort zone. Even trained doctors, nurses, counsellors, family therapists and rehabilitation workers can experience discomfort when sexual issues surface in the helping relationship with adults.[1-3] So what then do professionals do when it comes to dealing with sexual issues with adolescents? Avoid? Blunder in, blushing furiously? Ask only cursory questions in the hopes that we don't have to 'go there'? Hesitate in asking anything in case we find ourselves in possession of child protection information that we don't want to have to report?

Young people are sexually active at an increasingly younger age. Sticking our heads in the sands and hoping that 'someone else will address the issue' is not only unhelpful but also possibly harmful. It's important that youth be given the opportunity to discuss sexuality. When we consider substance use and the impact it can have on impulsivity, decision-making and the lowering of inhibition, educating ourselves and exploring sexual health with teenagers who use drugs is vital. In this chapter, we will examine the possible risks inherent when sexuality and substance use are mixed, as well as the substance use-related sexual issues that may need to be addressed.

SEX AND ADOLESCENCE

Our bodies begin changing from child to adult during adolescence. It is a time marked by rapid physiological change and development.[4] During puberty, young people's bodies force them to recognise their sexuality: breasts develop, periods commence, ejaculation occurs. According to the World Health Organization, adolescence is marked by sexual changes.[5] They suggest that sexual arousal increases and sexual behaviours commence, including masturbation, and same-sex or opposite-sex experimentation. Alongside these physical and sexual changes, teenagers grapple with a myriad of developmental milestones, social learning and the struggle for independence. This period in development can be linked with feelings of doubt, confusion, anger and upset, and that's before substance use is thrown in the mix. Questions about sexual orientation sometimes emerge at this time. Burgeoning sexual feelings and early sexual experiences are a normal part of development. Furthermore, unlike previous generations, young people today are increasingly exposed to sexuality. Television shows aimed at teenagers frequently have storylines centring on having sex, and nudity or near nudity is a common occurrence in movies and popular television. Popular music is littered with a multitude of sexual references, from the subtle to the outright crude. Gone are the days of parents flicking the television channel over when two characters in a show start kissing.

With changes in the media and social media, our young people are familiar with sexual issues at a much younger age. But just when exactly are our young people starting their voyage into sexual exploration? And when should we begin discussing it with them? Research into the sexual behaviours of Irish teens has shown that, despite the legal age of consent being 17, approximately one in five will have had sex before the age of 16.[6–8] The rates in the United States appear higher, with 47.4% of high school students reporting having had sex.[9] In a survey of 40 countries, Britain has the third-highest rate of sexual activity in teenagers aged between 13 and 15, with 32% stating they were sexually active.[10] In Australia, 44% of males and 67% of females report having had sex by the time they reach the twelfth grade (approximately 17 years old). Research tells us that no matter what way we look at it, many people are engaging in sexual activity before adulthood. As professionals, we can't ignore this. We need to address our own reluctance to explore these issues with adolescents, and educating ourselves is the best way forwards. Even if teenagers are not having sex they can still be involved in considerable sexual activity. A preliminary report in the UK[11] highlights the practice of teenagers distributing naked or sexually explicit pictures and videos of themselves via mobile phone and Internet sites. Naturally, these images can be potentially disastrous for the teenager.

LEGAL ISSUES

Perhaps one reason professionals avoid questions of a sexual nature is the minefield of legal and ethical issues it opens up. One area that causes much concern is that of consent. The age of consent varies from country to country.

Ultimately, professionals are faced with a dilemma. What happens when routine assessments garner information about sexual behaviour? What do we do if adolescents ask for contraceptives before they're legally allowed to have sex? How do we balance the need to adhere to the law *and* ensure young

TABLE 14.1 Age of consent in various countries

Country	Age of consent (years)
UK	16
Ireland	17
United States	16–18, depending on the state
Australia	16–18, depending on which state and what sexual act
Germany	14, with some restrictions applying
Italy	14, but 13-year-olds can consent to sex with someone up to 3 years older than their age
Spain	16 (raised from 13 in 2013)

people who choose to have sex before the age of consent minimise the risk of unplanned pregnancy or a sexually transmitted infection (STI)?

In the UK, the 'Fraser guidelines' ensure professionals can give under-16s advice about contraceptives and treatment under strict conditions. Technically, if a professional in Ireland learns that a young person is having sex under the age of consent, he or she is supposed to report it to social workers. In reality, social workers are unlikely to respond to two 16-year-olds having consensual sex, but the damage to the relationship between the teenager and worker may already be done. The impact on the therapeutic relationship may be that the young person feels betrayed. Ethical dilemmas don't tend to have simple solutions and it's important to seek consultation when faced with such issues. Forester-Miller and Davis[12] suggest the following as a model for making ethical decisions:

- identify the problem
- apply your professional code of ethics
- determine the nature and dimensions of the dilemma
- generate potential courses of action
- consider the potential consequences of all options; choose a course of action
- evaluate the selected course of action
- implement the course of action.

Seeking consultation with your colleagues, reviewing the literature, clarifying what is or isn't happening, considering the worst-case scenario and asking yourself if you would be happy if your decision were published are also strategies you can use to help make these decisions. It's not easy, but we have to put the health and welfare of young people above our own reluctance to make decisions. Not asking questions that we suspect may bring forth answers that straddle the boundaries of ethical and legal issues is not good practice.

Ultimately, the primary responsibility of the worker is to the minor. Educate yourself. Familiarise yourself with the range of sexual issues that may be present with adolescent substance use and the law and be a person who creates an environment where the young person feels safe to talk.

SEX AND SUBSTANCE USE IN ADOLESCENCE

While experimentation with substances and the move towards sexual expression can be part of adolescence, mixing the two can have complications. Later, we will examine the links between risky sexual behaviour and substance use in adolescents. First, it's important to note that not all of this risky behaviour is an unwitting consequence of mixing the two. Some adolescents have a clear-cut, strategic motivation for using substances in sexual situations. We've all heard the expression 'Dutch courage.' Well, now the evidence backs it up. One European study found that one-third of male and nearly a quarter of female adolescents reported using alcohol with the explicit purpose of facilitating a sexual encounter. Essentially, some of our young people are intentionally using alcohol when they want to have sex. Cocaine, cannabis and ecstasy were also reported as drugs used to prolong sex, enhance sexual feelings and increase arousal.[13]

Substance use has been linked to sexual risk behaviour in many studies, with substance use and the initiation of sexual activity closely linked.[14] Studies relating to onset of sexual activity and alcohol use in French, New Zealand, Scottish, English and European young people have all found a relationship between alcohol and early onset of sexual activity.[13,15,16] One study found that individuals were significantly more likely to have had sex before the age of 16 if they had used certain drugs before 16.[13] In an Irish study, substance use wasn't found to be a factor in sexual debut among adolescents; that being said, 30% of the respondents in this study reported that they had been under the influence at their first experience of intercourse.[6]

An American study found that more than a quarter (29%) of 15- to 17-year-old respondents reported that their substance use had influenced their decisions about sex, stating that they had 'done more' than they planned while under the influence of substances.[17] Twelve percent of the 15- to 17-year-olds reported having unprotected sex while drinking or using.[17] The findings related to poor sexual decision-making while under the influences and are corroborated in other studies that suggest substance use is related to indiscriminate forms of risky sexual behaviour.[18,19] A study exploring substance use and associated health risks across Europe found that cannabis, cocaine or ecstasy use was linked to higher numbers of sexual partners in the past month, unprotected sex and regretting having sex.[13] For professionals, helping clients deal with the practicalities and the feelings that may result from poor decision-making is important.

One of the darker sides of adolescent substance use is that of prostitution, not all of which occurs on street corners. In clinical practice, young girls sometimes share stories of 'sleeping with guys' they know have drugs, or staying with a partner simply because that partner provides access to substances. While they don't use words like prostitution, they describe a link between their sexual behaviour and the obtainment of substances. Research supports this: exchange of sex for drugs has been strongly linked to regular cocaine and ecstasy use, with more than one in seven regular ecstasy users having done so in the past year.[13] Feelings of shame, guilt and self-loathing can accompany these disclosures, and in some cases these feelings act as a trigger to use more substances.

Ecstasy, 'the love drug', is one that is much discussed in relation to sexual behaviour. In reality, research on the matter is inconclusive. Most studies on the effects of ecstasy suggest users experience feelings of closeness, sensuality and empathy while under the influence. Other studies have found that it does indeed increase sexual arousal in users. Interestingly, most respondents in one study reported feelings of closeness without the desire for penetrative sex but other respondents in the same study had used ecstasy for sexual enhancement.[20] In this study, sexual risk-taking was rife among those who engaged in sexual behaviour while under the influence. This included unprotected sex and engaging in sexual behaviour with multiple partners. Interestingly, despite its infamy as the love drug, many studies on ecstasy have discovered that it can be associated with sexual impairment.[21,22]

Another consideration is unplanned pregnancy. Studies have found a correlation between alcohol-related hospital admissions and teenage pregnancy.[23,24] Condom use appears to be an issue when alcohol forms part of the picture regarding sexual activity. Those under the influence at their first sexual encounter appear less likely to use condoms than those who aren't drinking.[25] This may be a factor in both rates of teen pregnancy and of STI transmission among younger clients.

Diagnoses of STIs among teenage alcohol users are high. In general, adolescents and young people represent almost 50% of all new STIs.[26] The US National Survey on Drug Use and Health found that young people who had used both alcohol and an illicit drug in the past month were more likely to have had an STI in the past year. STI rates among those who use alcohol but not drugs were also higher than in a comparable group who used neither.

Given these research findings on the possible links between adolescent substance use, STIs and teen pregnancy, it is vital that we educate ourselves about these issues. Remember, education is key to reducing professionals' discomfort about discussing sexual issues.

SEXUALLY TRANSMITTED INFECTIONS

There are more than 30 different sexually transmissible bacteria, viruses and parasites, but only 19 are named as the main causative agents of STIs.[27,28] In the UK, rates of STIs are highest among those in their twenties, followed by those in the 15- to 19-year age range.[29] While it would be impossible to describe them all in this chapter, we will discuss in the following section some of the STIs common among adolescents. We also discuss the human immunodeficiency virus (HIV) and the hepatitis C virus (HCV), which drug users are at an increased risk of contracting. More information is available through the website of the US Centers for Disease Control and Prevention (www.cdc.gov).

Chlamydia

Chlamydia remains the most common STI among young people in England. This trend continues in Ireland, where chlamydia is the most prevalent infection among those in their twenties, accounting for 69.8% of STI notifications.[29,30]

Chlamydia can be transmitted during anal, oral or vaginal sex or from mother to baby. It is known as the 'silent' STI, as many people have no symptoms. For women who do experience symptoms, abnormal discharge, a burning sensation while urinating, back pain, bleeding between periods and fever are the most common. Men can experience discharge from their penis and pain while urinating. For those who engage in anal sex, there can be rectal pain, discharge or bleeding. Chlamydia can lead to serious reproductive health consequences such as pelvic inflammatory disease, infertility, ectopic pregnancies and problems with the reproductive organs.[4,31] The good news is that treatment is a simple course of antibiotics. It's important to catch it early, as the longer it goes untreated, the higher the risk of long-term consequences. A simple test can be conducted in any genito-urinary clinic and some GP clinics. In fact, home test kits are available in many pharmacies.

Genital warts

The human papillomavirus is the most commonly diagnosed STI in sexual health clinics around the world. There are many different strains of this virus and not everyone who contracts it will develop genital warts. For those who do develop warts, there is usually a gap of between 1 and 3 months from the date of infection to when the warts appear.[4] The symptoms include small cauliflower-shaped lumps on the genital area. They can appear on the vagina, anus, penis, vulva and into the cervix. Treatment for genital warts consists of the application of a cream, liquid or chemical directly onto the warts. Another treatment option is where the warts are cut, burned off or removed with a laser.[32]

Gonorrhoea

Gonorrhoea, sometimes referred to as 'the clap', is caused by a bacterium that is transmitted through penetrative sex, sharing sex toys or touching infected sex parts. It can be passed from mother to baby. Like chlamydia, it is possible to be asymptomatic, but women may experience a strong-smelling discharge that changes colour to a yellowish green, pain when urinating and irritation of the anus. Men can also experience discharge from the penis and inflammation of the prostate and testicles. Treatment is a course of antibiotics. It is important to get treatment, as it can lead to problems with fertility and ectopic pregnancy if left untreated.

Human immunodeficiency virus

By the end of 2009, an estimated 33 million people in the world were living with HIV. The human immunodeficiency virus is the virus that causes acquired immune deficiency syndrome (AIDS). The virus attacks the body's T-cells, which are required to fight infections. HIV is transmitted through the sharing of sexual fluids or blood. Unprotected oral, anal or vaginal sex and the sharing of needles are common ways in which it's transmitted. Once it was known as the 'gay man's disease', but in recent years, heterosexual sex became the most common route of transmission.[4] Drug users are at an increased risk, not only those who inject but also those who engage in sexual activity with intravenous drug users. Injecting drug use has directly and indirectly accounted for more than one-third (36%) of AIDS cases in the United States.[33,34] There is no cure for HIV but strides have been made in the treatment. It is no longer the death sentence it once was, with over 30 retroviral medications in use today. While these drugs don't eradicate the virus, they act as suppressors, and in some cases they suppress it to undetectable levels. This means longer and healthier lives are now possible.

HIV has a window period of 3 months. Essentially, this means that it can take 3 months after sexual contact with an infected partner for the virus to show up in your blood. During this time and, indeed, for a long time after infection, no symptoms may be present. Even those who do experience symptoms can put it down to a bad flu. Therefore, waiting on the appearance of symptoms is not a reliable way to diagnose. Screening for HIV involves a blood test. Anyone who has had unprotected sex is at risk and it is advisable to get tested.

Needle exchange clinics are an important tool in the fight against the spread of HIV. Of course, in an ideal world there would be no need for us to refer young people to such services, but we don't live in an ideal world. Harm reduction might not sit well with some workers, but it *is* necessary. It is far better that an adolescent has access to clean needles and using paraphernalia than they contract HIV as a result of poor using practice.

Hepatitis C

HCV is most commonly transmitted through the sharing of injecting drug use paraphernalia. Across the world, 90% of all new HCV diagnoses are attributed to injecting drug use. Approximately half of all injecting drug users in the UK have HCV.[29] In Ireland, the prevalence among injecting drug users attending community-based drug services range between 52% and 84%.[35] In Australia, 90% of HCV cases are contracted through intravenous drug use.[36] Sex with multiple partners and prostitution are also linked to hepatitis infection.[4] The symptoms of HCV include tiredness, flu-like symptoms, stomach upset, joint pain, weight loss and jaundice. In severe cases, it can lead to liver and brain damage. There are different strains of the virus and it is possible to have more than one strain at a time. In 25% of cases, the body will naturally eliminate the virus, but for the other 75%, treatment is sometimes necessary. This consists of the use of antiviral medication.

Again, educating clients about safe injecting practice and the presence of local needle exchanges is important. While the risk for sexual transmission isn't as high, it is still present; therefore, it's *always* advisable to encourage use of condoms when engaging in sexual activity with a drug-using partner.

SEXUAL CONSEQUENCES OF SUBSTANCE USE

While we saw earlier that some young people intentionally use substances to heighten arousal, substance use can have a devastating effect on sexual functioning. Alcohol, cocaine, opiates and amphetamines can all contribute to erectile dysfunction.[37] Likewise, illicit drug use has also been found to inhibit sexual desire.[38]

Anecdotally, cocaine users report heightened sex drive and enjoyable sexual experiences while under the influence. In reality, cocaine use has been linked to erectile dysfunction, sexual desire disorders, infertility and compulsive sexual behaviours. Whatever short-term sexual satisfaction accompanies cocaine, its use can be associated with a myriad of nasty and sometimes persistent sexual problems. For women, cocaine use can have a long-term effect on their ovulation cycle, and for men, it has been associated with low sperm count.

Heroin also affects sexual functioning. For women who use opiates, it is not uncommon for their menstrual cycle to become irregular or even stop completely. Women struggle to orgasm and men routinely fail to ejaculate. A decrease in libido and an overall change in sexual behaviour are evident in those who use heroin.[39] While many people see cannabis as a drug of lesser evil, it too could have implications for sexual functioning. While research is contradictory, one recent study suggests that it may have a negative effect on erectile function in men.[40]

So while young people may choose to use substances to initiate or heighten sexual experiences, they may be blissfully unaware of the long-term sexual consequences to the behaviour they are choosing.

TALKING TO YOUNG PEOPLE ABOUT SEX

Most youth services will be aware of the importance of assessment. Often during an assessment process, we will explore a range of areas of functioning with the young person. It's routine in many services to obtain a full history, including family, developmental, social and substance use history. Emotional well-being and vocational and education history might also be included. Young people are sexual creatures and many are engaging in sexual activity. When substance use forms part of this picture, this sexual activity may be high risk. Now, ask yourself this question: Does our service routinely ask about sexual history? If not, why not?

When asked about having discussions about sexual issues, young people prefer that workers adopt a supportive, welcoming, understanding but professional way of being. The importance of confidentiality, being treated like an adult and getting straight answers were also highlighted.[41,42] This means we need to be able to discuss these issues in a straight and forthright manner. Take a moment to reflect on that. How comfortable are you discussing these issues? Making exploration of sexual issues a part of routine practice can go a long way to helping young people manage their sexual health. Adopt a matter-of-fact, professional approach to assessment, interviewing, information giving and referral. Also, by assessing sexual issues regularly, staff will become more skilled and relaxed in discussing sexual issues.

CONCLUSIONS

As we have seen, sexuality is an important aspect of adolescent development. Many teenagers are sexually active, often despite national laws forbidding their behaviour. Substance-using adolescents are probably more likely to be sexually active and their activities also tend to be more risky (e.g. unprotected sex). In order to limit the harm related to their sexual activity assessment is vital. Those who are sexually active should be encouraged to use condoms and undergo regular screening for STIs.

KEY POINTS
- Education is paramount to reducing a professional's discomfort about exploring sexual issues.

- Young people can use substances intentionally when they approach sexual situations.
- Substance use is linked to teen pregnancy, higher rates of STIs, regretted sex, multiple sex partners, poor contraceptive use and a range of high-risk sexual behaviours.
- STI rates are high among adolescent substance users. Familiarise yourself with local genito-urinary clinics.
- Substance use has been linked to problems in sexual functioning.

FURTHER READING

➡ Public Health England and the NHS' website provides a wealth of information on a variety of health topics including sexual health. www.nhs.uk/sexualhealth

REFERENCES

1 Juergens MH, Smedena SM, Berven NL. Willingness of graduate students in rehabilitation counselling to discuss sexuality with clients. *Rehabil Couns Bull.* 2009; **53**(1): 34–43.

2 Harris SM, Hays KW. Family therapist comfort with and willingness to discuss client sexuality. *J Marital Fam Ther.* 2008; **34**(2): 239–50.

3 Gott M, Galena E, Hinchliff S, *et al.* 'Open a can of worms': GP and practice nurse barriers to talking about sexual health in primary care. *Fam Pract.* 2004; **21**(5): 528–36.

4 Bekaert S. *Adolescents and Sex: the handbook for professionals working with young people.* Oxford: Radcliffe Publishing; 2005.

5 World Health Organization (WHO). *Counselling Skills Training in Adolescent Sexuality and Reproductive Health.* Geneva: WHO; 2001.

6 Hyde A, Howlett E. *Understanding Teenage Sexuality in Ireland.* Dublin: Crisis Pregnancy Agency; 2004.

7 Bonner C. A *Report on the Sexual Practices of 16–18 year olds in the Midland Health Board.* Department of Public Health, Midland Health Board; 1996.

8 Lalor K, O'Regan C, Quinlan S. Determinants of sexual behaviour. *Irish J Sociol.* 2003; **12**(2): 121–33.

9 Centers for Disease Control and Prevention (CDC). Trends in HIV-related risk behaviors among high school students: United States, 1991–2011. *MMWR Morb Mortal Wkly Rep.* 2012; **61**(29): 556–60.

10 Patton GG, Coffey C, Cappa C, *et al.* Health of the world's adolescents: a synthesis of internationally comparable data. *Lancet.* 2012; **379**(9826): 1665–75.

11 Phippen A. *Sexting: an exploration of practices, attitudes and influences.* UK Safer Internet Centre; 2012. Available at: www.saferinternet.org.uk/downloads/News/Sexting_An_Exploration_of_Practices_Attitudes_and_Influences_.pdf (accessed 1 January 2013).

12 Forester-Miller H, Davis T. *A Practitioner's Guide to Ethical Decision Making.* Alexandria, VA: American Counseling Association; 1996.

13 Bellis M, Hughes K, Calafat A, *et al.* Sexual uses of alcohol and drugs and the associated health risks: a cross sectional study of young people in nine European cities. *BMC Public Health.* 2008; **8**(1): 155.

14 Mott FL, Haurin RJ. Linkages between sexual activity and alcohol and drug use among American adolescents. *Fam Plann Perspect.* 1988; **20**(3): 128–36.

15 Choquet M, Manfredi R. Sexual intercourse, contraception, and risk-taking behavior among unselected French adolescents aged 11–20 years. *J Adolesc Health.* 1992; **13**(7): 623–30.

16 Fergusson DM, Lynskey MT. Alcohol misuse and adolescent sexual behaviors and risk taking. *Pediatrics.* 1996; **98**(1): 91–6.

17 Kaiser Family Foundation. *National Survey of Youth Knowledge and Attitudes on Sexual Health Issues.* Menlo Park, CA: Kaiser Family Foundation; 2002.

18 Cooper ML. Alcohol use and risky sexual behaviour among college students and youth: evaluating the evidence. *J Stud Alcohol Suppl.* 2002; (14): 101–17.

19 Senf JH, Price CQ. Young adults, alcohol and condom use: what is the connection? *J Adolesc Health.* 1994; **15**(3): 238–44.

20 McElrath K. MDMA and sexual behaviour: Ecstasy users' perceptions about sexuality and sexual risk. *Subst Use Misuse.* 2005; **40**(9–10): 1461–77.

21 Zeimishlany Z, Aizenberg D, Weizman A. Subjective effects of MDMA (Ecstasy) on human sexual function. *Eur Psychiatry.* 2001; **16**(2): 127–30.

22 Passie T, Hartmann U, Schneider U, *et al.* Ecstasy (MDMA) mimics the post-orgasmic state: impairment of sexual drive and function during acute MDMA-effects may be due to increased prolactin secretion. *Med Hypotheses.* 2005; **64**(5): 899–903.

23 Bellis MA, Morleo M, Tocque K, *et al. Contributions of Alcohol Use to Teenage Pregnancy: an initial examination of geographical and evidence based associations.* Liverpool: Liverpool John Moores University; 2009.

24 Cook PA, Harkins C, Morleo, M, *et al. Contributions of Alcohol Use to Teenage Pregnancy and Sexually Transmitted Infection Rates.* Liverpool: Liverpool John Moores University; 2010.

25 Leigh BC. Alcohol and condom use: a meta-analysis of event-level studies. *Sex Transm Dis.* 2002; **29**(8): 476–82.

26 Da Ros CT, Schmitt CD. Global epidemiology of sexually transmitted diseases. *Asian J Androl.* 2008; **10**(1): 110–14.

27 Chinembu KC. Sexually transmitted infections in adolescents. *Open Infect Dis J.* 2009; **3**: 107–17.

28 Word Health Organization (WHO). *Global Strategy for the Prevention and Control of Sexually Transmitted Infections 2006–2015.* Geneva: WHO; 2007.

29 Health Protection Agency. *Hepatitis C in the UK.* London: Health Protection Agency; 2011.

30 Health Protection Surveillance Centre. *Sexually Transmitted Infections (STIs) & HIV in Ireland.* Dublin: Health Service Executive; 2008.

31 Centers for Disease Control and Prevention (CDC). *Chlamydia-CDC Fact Sheet.* Rockville, MD: CDC; 2012.

32 National Health Service (NHS). *Genital Warts: treatment.* NHS Choices; 2012. Available at: www.nhs.uk/Conditions/Genital_warts/Pages/Treatment.aspx (accessed 11 August 2013).

33 Centers for Disease Control and Prevention (CDC). *HIV/AIDS Surveillance Report, 2007.* Vol. 19. Atlanta, GA: US Department of Health and Human Services; 2007.

34 Centers for Disease Control and Prevention (CDC). *HIV/AIDS.* Atlanta, GA: CDC; 2009. Available at: www.cdc.gov/hiv/topics/surveillance/resources/reports/ (accessed 11 August 2013).

35 Hellard M, Sacks-Davis R, Gold J. Hepatitis C treatment for injection drug users: a review of the available evidence. *Clin Infect Dis.* 2009; **49**(4): 561–73.

36 Long J. Epidemiology of hepatitis C among drug users in Ireland. *Drugnet Ireland.* 2004; **11**: 8–10.

37 Hepatitis C, Virus Projections Working Group. *Estimates and Projections of the Hepatitis C Virus Epidemic in Australia 2006.* Canberra: Hepatitis C Sub-Committee, Ministerial Advisory Committee on AIDS Sexual Health and Hepatitis; 2006.

38 Jiann BP. Erectile dysfunction associated with psychoactive substances. *Chonnam Med J.* 2008; **44**(3): 117–24.

39 Hales RE, Yudofsky SC, Gabbard GO, editors. *Textbook of Psychiatry.* 5th ed. Arlington, VA: American Psychiatric Publishing; 2008.

40 Zharkov Y. Sexuality of heroin addicts. *Eur J Med Sexol.* 2002; **11**(39): 33–44.

41 Shamioul R, Bella AJ. The impact of cannabis use on male sexual health. *J Sex Med.* 2011; **8**(4): 971–5.

42 Mitchell K, Wellings K. *Talking about Sexual Health.* London: Health Education Authority; 1998.

CHAPTER 15

Substance use and cultural issues

INTRODUCTION

Difference can be challenging. Individuals are drawn to settle in groups where a common sense of identity is shared. Our roots are set down in a shared culture and the challenges of accepting one another's race and ethnicity have been played out over time from nation to nation. Migration brings the opportunity to interact with and learn about other cultures, customs and experiences. It also brings the possibility of misunderstanding and prejudice. However, culture is not limited to the shared identity of the country in which we were born or our ethnicity. Indeed, groups of people born in the same country or town and of the same race can have very different cultural backgrounds.

Children and young people, ethnic minorities and the travelling community are three of the six groups identified in Ireland's *National Action Plan for Social Inclusion 2007–2016*[1] as being at increased risk of social exclusion. Young people have their own culture and subcultures. Anyone who has watched even one teen movie will have seen the stereotypical Hollywood delineation of subculture within a school setting. Cheerleaders will sit at one table while the studious gather together at another; adolescents dressed in black, with dark lipstick, nail polish, eye make-up and dark hair will congregate at yet another table. There is little interaction between these groups, and each will have their own musical taste, dress sense and sets of beliefs. Here in one room, in one town, in one country, we can see how subculture plays out.

When working with adolescents, skills, knowledge and awareness are needed to enable practitioners to become culturally competent. In this chapter, we will examine definitions of culture and explore some of the competencies required to work effectively with diversity.

DEFINITIONS

While increasing volumes have been written about multiculturalism and diversity in recent years, many authors do not clarify what they understand by the various terms. In this section, we will offer readers a definition of both culture and multiculturalism.

Culture

> The terms 'culture' and 'cultural' are used to refer to the customs, attitudes, experiences and/or traditions that may be shared (or disputed) by groups of people, through belonging to particular national or ethnic groups.[2]

Jewsebury, *et al.*'s[2] definition clearly shows that culture comprises a variety of social factors. Nelson-Jones,[3] citing Spindler, offers another useful definition of culture when he says that culture is 'a pattern system of tradition-derived norms influencing behaviour.' Nelson-Jones[3] offers a wonderful colloquial definition of culture when he describes it as 'the way we do things here.'

If we consider the root of the word culture – to cultivate – we can see that these factors aren't built; they grow. We learn them as we grow in our families, our education systems, and our peer groups. Culture is something that can and does change.

Subculture

According to *The Concise Oxford Dictionary*,[4] a subculture is:

> A cultural group within a larger culture, often having beliefs or interests at variance with those of the larger culture.

There are a myriad of subcultures evident in adolescent society. Furthermore, there can be a variety of subcultures evident among substance-using teenagers. Those who use cannabis may have different beliefs, behaviours and attitudes to those who use heroin. Society may view drugs users as one homogenous group; however, within that group, varied subcultures exist who may not identify with one another in any way.

Multiculturalism

Jewsebury, *et al.*[2] suggest that multi- and interculturalism are sometimes used interchangeably and purport that this is inaccurate. Multiculturalism is the coexistence of several cultures in the same nation. Interculturalism suggests that many cultures not only exist together but also mix together, for the greater part harmoniously.

While nations are understood to share a common culture there are many cultural subgroups within seemingly homogenous groups. Indeed, individual families develop unique family subcultures within their culture. We each have different ways of marking birthdays or not, of sharing family time or not.

CULTURAL ISSUES IN SUBSTANCE USE

Social inclusion in service provision for adolescent substance misuse emphasises the need to offer care to adolescents who experience a range of social differences. Young people present from a range of different ethnic groups, sexual orientations and cultural backgrounds.

According to Gordan,[5]

> cultural competence is essential in acquiring the trust of ethnic minority clients and ethnic communities, as well as in understanding the ways different cultural groups define health . . . especially in relation to substance use.

This means that practitioners have an obligation to become culturally competent. So how do we do this? Burnham, *et al.*[6] provide us with a very useful framework for developing cultural competencies. They describe social differences that are encountered and they invite us to become aware of our own perceptions of this diversity. This chapter will explore Burnham, *et al.*'s[6] 'Social GRRAACCEESS' and present reflections on some of them in the context of adolescent substance misuse (*see* Box 15.1).

BOX 15.1 Social GRRAACCEESS[6]

G = Gender
R = Race
R = Religion
A = Age
A = Ability(Dis)
C = Culture
C = Class
E = Education
E = Ethnicity
S = Sexual orientation
S = Spirituality

While it isn't possible in this chapter to explore them all, we encourage you to reflect on each of them and how they might influence your practice and interactions with young people. Do you have any particular biases? Are there gaps in your knowledge? What are the possible implications of proceeding in your attempts to help an adolescent substance user with a different culture to your own without the necessary information about their culture?

Now let's take a look at a few headings Burnham, *et al.*[6] propose in the Social GRRAACCEESS framework and consider them from a substance use perspective.

Gender

Gender is an important factor in how people experience the world around them. It can influence their roles and behaviours, and the opportunities they encounter.[7] Gender issues must be considered when it comes to adolescent substance use. Engaging young people in a supporting process can be difficult. A recent study into adult therapy retention rates found that 'rates of dropout were highest among the youngest participants.'[8] Dropout rates are also higher among males.[9] Research suggests that males report substance use more than their female counterparts.[10] The authors of a report published in 2004 suggest that 'pathways to substance use are different for men and women and these differences impact the decision to seek treatment, remain in treatment, and the ability to achieve successful outcomes.'[10]

In our own practice, we certainly see more adolescent males presenting for treatment than females; however, of note is the level of psychological distress that female clients present with. In a 2010 study, we found that girls with a SUD (substance use disorder) 'differ from their male counterparts in having both more internalizing and externalizing psychiatric problems.'[11] Essentially, females are more likely to exhibit symptoms of internal psychological distress, such as depression and anxiety, *and* external disorders such as behavioural problems. This finding is noteworthy when we consider that male adolescents are far more likely to encounter legal consequences as a result of their drug use behaviour. One has to ask if perhaps female substance users are given more leniencies in the judicial system.

Another factor to consider is that up to 70% of female substance abusers have a history of child sexual abuse.[12] Female clients may be more likely to present with symptoms of trauma, and, as such, they may be more likely to relapse.[13] This has implications in terms of treatment and suggests that those directly involved in substance abuse treatment need to have a good understanding of child sexual abuse. This is important also for those working with young people in general. If a client is substance using, it may be an indication that there are complex issues at play that may require referral to specialist services.

Psychological health is not the only facet worth reflecting on. Lim[14] suggests that while female problem drinkers consume less alcohol than males, they develop serious health issues like cirrhosis and cardiomyopathy at a quicker rate than men. Tuchman[15] contends that we also need to be aware of 'gender-specific medical problems'. She goes on to suggest that women are more at risk of acquiring HIV as a result of their 'drug use patterns and sex-related risk behaviours.'[15]

Religion

As described in Chapter 5, involvement in religion can be a protective factor against substance use, but it's also important to consider the cultural implications of religion when working with young people who use substances. Beliefs about substance use can vary from faith to faith. In some religions, drugs are used for spiritual purposes, while in others they are completely prohibited.

For example, while the Catholic Church doesn't forbid the use of alcohol, drunkenness and drug use is not looked upon favourably. Clients raised in a strict Catholic background may also experience strong feelings of guilt following a night out where their substance use facilitated the engagement in unplanned sexual activity. Other religious groups are opposed to any use of alcohol or drugs. The Church of the Jesus Christ of Latter-Day Saints has a strict moral code that includes abstinence from alcohol, nicotine and illicit drugs. Members who don't adhere to this are unable to participate fully in the activities of the church and can find themselves isolated from their community while they engage in drug-using behaviour. Muslims also abstain from alcohol and drugs and we have worked with some Middle Eastern Muslims who are dealing with the additional worry of prison or other severe punishments should their substance use be revealed.

Now, consider a client who presents from a religious background where abstinence is a requirement. The need for secrecy about his or her substance use may be hugely important. As professionals, we understand that family involvement is correlated with better outcomes, but what do we do when we know that involving family members may further isolate the client from the potentially protective factor of his or her religion and family?

Shame may be present in the young person who was raised in a religious culture where substance misuse is abhorred. What might be happening for the teenager whose external behaviour of drug use is completely incongruent with his or her internal religious beliefs? Reflect on what it might be like to live with that internal conflict. Like any facet of culture, it's important to seek an understanding of our client's religious beliefs and background. If a client presents from a religion that is unfamiliar to you, read up and research it. Awareness and knowledge help to avoid misunderstandings. There may be aspects of your clients' religious beliefs that could support them in trying to make changes.

Class

There is an expectation that drug misuse is the preserve of disadvantaged communities. This can create dilemmas on all sides. Parents, families and schools in middle- and upper-class communities may be less vigilant for drug misuse and its indicators. While middle- and upper-class families can more easily provide many of the protective factors for drug and alcohol misuse, class cannot be seen as an inoculation against substance misuse problems.

When families in more privileged positions find that their son or daughter is having difficulties with substance use, parents often become isolated. They may feel that this should not be happening and can go to great lengths to manage the situation without any support. They hesitate to confide in family members, as they want to protect the reputation of their child. Yet in this they can begin to collude with the difficulties that are dominating their lives. Likewise, young people from disadvantaged areas may be more likely to face challenges such as parental substance use, poverty, lower educational attainment and lack of resources.

Ethnicity

Lim[14] purports that different ethnic backgrounds can have different substance use treatment issues and we should assist them to draw on their own cultural strengths when we consider treatment planning. Thus, it is important to familiarise ourselves with our clients' cultural norms. For example, in many Western cultures, maintaining eye contact when speaking to someone is the norm. In fact, we may view poor eye contact in a therapeutic space as an attempt to avoid connection. However, in many cultures it is deemed disrespectful. In fact, in some countries women won't make eye contact with men at all in case it is interpreted as a sexual overture. Cultural norms around other non-verbal behaviours such as gesticulation and touch may also vary.[16]

Reflection

How might you deal with a client from a different country who presents to your service for support but who doesn't make eye contact, despite your repeated attempts to engage with him or her? Can you accept and understand that this may actually be a sign of respect? Do you immediately make a judgement based on your cultural norm? Likewise, if you're from a culture where maintaining eye contact is not the norm, how might you deal with adolescents who expect you will look at them when they are talking to you?

In some cultures, such as those of the Australian Aborigines, people don't speak the name of deceased loved ones. This is quite different from Western cultures, where the person is 'waked' and we are encouraged to talk about the person, sharing our memories. Neither custom is better than the other; they are simply different. The important thing for professionals is to remember we need to find a way of helping that is acceptable to the cultural norms of the client. Our way is not the only way, nor is it necessarily the right way. It is simply, as Nelson-Jones[3] put it, 'the way we do things round here.' Just remember that 'the way we do things' may not suit every client. As professionals we have an obligation to work with all clients, and to do this effectively we need to inform and educate ourselves around their cultural norms.

Sexual orientation

Research into rates of substance use and substance use disorder among lesbian, gay and bisexual (LGB) adolescents suggest that this client group are more likely to use substances than their heterosexual counterparts.[17,18] However, perhaps this is a simple statistic that can be easily misinterpreted. Being LGB in and of itself may not be a risk factor for substance use, but in a society that can still be largely homophobic and heterosexist, LGB clients can face added isolation, discrimination, bullying and alienation, which can all contribute to the person choosing drug or alcohol use to escape the pain.[19] Minority stress can be an additional consideration.

Likewise, internalised homophobia can play a part. If an LGB young person has been reared in a family that condemns homosexuality, that young person may grow up with the belief that there is something wrong with him or her. We live in a society that can send out negative messages about homosexuality – even the LGB young person raised in a supportive family environment internalises the negative messages of society. Imagine for a moment what it might be like to live with that conflict. To know you are gay, but to have the belief that there is something wrong with you.

A lack of culturally competent services adds to the problem. We live in a heterosexist world. How often have you seen an ad for a romantic getaway that featured a same-sex couple? How many times have you heard a female singer croon a love song to her girlfriend? Probably not too often! Music, advertising, television and radio is primarily heterosexist, and this can be true, too, of many support services.

While written for psychologists, the British Psychological Society and the American Psychological Association provide guidelines on any therapeutic practice with LGB clients.[20,21] They suggest that we try to comprehend the impact of negative attitudes towards homosexuality and bisexuality – the violence and stigmatisation that can occur. We are encouraged to leave behind the historical view that homosexuality is a mental disorder and to, instead, embrace homosexuality as a variant of human sexuality. The guidelines are too comprehensive to explore in this chapter, but they are worth a read for any practitioner who works with LGB clients.[20,21]

Reflection

Take a moment to consider your place of work. Are your health promotion posters LGB friendly? Are there leaflets about LGB resources freely displayed? Do your assessment forms ask about relationship status or marital status? When a client refers to his or her partner, would you ask if the partner is male or female or would you just assume the opposite gender to your client? Do you have an understanding of the coming-out process? Are you comfortable discussing sexual issues that are perhaps different to your sexual norms?

CONCLUSION

As we saw earlier in this chapter, culture is not a fixed entity. We grow, learn and adapt all the time. Our beliefs are changeable and challengeable. In order to become more culturally competent, we are encouraged to consider the following[22]:

- increase your understanding and knowledge around diversity
- recognise that culture is an important aspect of psychological processes
- professionals should have an awareness of both their own and their client's cultural background
- respect the client's culture and the values inherent within it
- consider the language barrier
- include the client's experiences of racism, sexism and homophobia when treatment planning or designing a care plan
- understand the influence that culture, gender, sexual orientation, race or class may have on the client's behaviours.

Ultimately, we challenge you to respect and embrace the diversity that presents in working with adolescents. You don't need to be an expert on every race or religion, but bear in mind the impact that culture can have on the relationship and on the client's outcome.

KEY POINTS

- Culture is a complex phenomenon and includes ethnicity, gender, sexuality, socio-economic, religious and other differences.
- Subcultures can exist between groups within society and can lead to considerable differences between teenagers.

• In order to provide client-centred care that is appropriate and sensitive to the needs of each individual, staff need to ensure they are knowledgeable of and give due regard to each client's individual circumstance.

FURTHER READING

➡ Pope-Davis DB, Coleman HLK. *Multicultural Counselling Competencies: assessment, education and training, and supervision.* London: Sage Publications; 1997.
➡ Jordon JU. *Managing Multiculturalism in Substance Abuse Services.* London: Sage Publications; 1994.

REFERENCES

1 Government of Ireland. *National Action Plan for Social Inclusion 2007–2016.* Dublin: The Stationery Office; 2007.
2 Jewsebury D, Singh J, Tuck S. *Cultural Diversity and the Arts Research Project: towards the development of an Arts Council policy and action plan.* Dublin: The Arts Council; 2009.
3 Nelson-Jones R. *The Theory and Practice of Counselling and Therapy.* 5th ed. London: Sage Publications; 2010.
4 Pearsall J, editor. *The Concise Oxford Dictionary.* 10th ed, revised. Oxford: Oxford University Press.
5 Gordon JU. *Managing Multiculturalism in Substance Abuse Services.* Thousand Oaks, CA: Sage Publications; 1994.
6 Burnham J, Alvis-Palma D, Whitehouse L. Learning as a context for differences and differences as a context for learning. *J Fam Ther.* 2008; **30**(4): 529–42.
7 Fassinger RE, Sperber-Richie B. Sex matters: gender and sexual orientation in training for multicultural counselling competency. In: Pope-Davis DB, Coleman HLK, editors. *Multicultural Counselling Competencies: assessment, education and training, and supervision.* London: Sage Publications; 1997. pp. 83–110.
8 Swift JK, Greenberg RP. Premature discontinuation in adult psychotherapy: a meta-analysis. *J Consult Clin Psychol.* 2012; **80**(4): 547–59.
9 Reneses B, Munoz E, Lópes-Ibor JJ. Factors predicting drop-out in community mental health centres. *World Psychiatry.* 2009; **8**(3): 173–7.
10 Office of Substance Abuse Services (OSAS). *Gender Differences and their Implications for Substance Use Disorder Treatment.* Virginia: OSAS; 2004.
11 Edokpolo O, James P, Kearns C, *et al.* Gender differences in psychiatric symptomatology in adolescents attending a community drug and alcohol treatment program. *J Psychoactive Drugs.* 2010; **42**(1): 31–6.
12 National Institute on Drug Abuse. Gender differences in drug abuse risks and treatment. *NIDA Notes.* 2000; **15**(4). Available at: http://archives.drugabuse.gov/NIDA_Notes/NNVol15N4/Tearoff.html (accessed 11 August 2013).
13 Brown PJ. Outcome in female patients with both substance use and post-traumatic stress disorders. *Alcohol Treat Q.* 2000; **18**(3): 127–35.

14 Lim RF. *Cultural Differences in Substance Abuse Treatment.* Presented at the 38th Semi-Annual Substance Abuse Research Consortium (SARC) Meeting; Sacramento, CA, 23 September 2008.

15 Tuchman E. Women and addiction: the importance of gender issues in substance abuse research. *J Addict Dis.* 2010; **29**(2): 127–38.

16 Vermont Department of Health. *Health Screen Recommendations for Children and Adolescents: cultural differences in non-verbal communication.* Burlington: Vermont Department of Health; 2011. Available at: http://healthvermont.gov/family/toolkit/ (accessed 11 August 2013).

17 Beatty RL, Madl R, Bostwick W. LGBT substance use. In: Shankle MD, editor. *Handbook of LGBT Public Health.* New York, NY: Haworth Press; 2004. pp. 201–20.

18 Marshal MQ. Sexual orientation and adolescent substance use: a meta-analysis and methodological review. *Addiction.* 2008; **103**(4): 546–56.

19 Centre for Addiction and Mental Health (CAMH). *Substance Use: issues to consider for the lesbian, gay, bisexual, transgendered, transsexual, two-spirit, intersex and queer communities.* Toronto: CAMH; 2012. Available at: www.ccsa.ca/Eng/Topics/Populations/LGBTTTIQ/Pages/default.aspx (accessed 11 August 2013).

20 American Psychological Association. Guidelines for psychological practice with lesbian, gay, and bisexual clients. *Am Psychol.* 2012; **67**(1): 10–42.

21 British Psychological Society. *Guidelines and Literature Review for Psychologists Working Therapeutically with Sexual and Gender Minority Clients.* Leicester: British Psychological Society; 2012.

22 Sodowsky GR, Kuo-Jackson PY, Loya GJ. Outcome of training in the philosophy of assessment: multicultural counselling competencies. In: Pope-Davis DB, Coleman HLK, editors. *Multicultural Counselling Competencies: assessment, education and training, and supervision.* London: Sage Publications; 1997. pp. 3–42.

CHAPTER 16

Inter-agency working

INTRODUCTION

Young people with various needs come into contact with a variety of professionals, including teachers, doctors and nurses. When teenagers struggle, even more professionals can become involved, including social workers, counsellors, psychologists, speech and language therapists and education welfare staff. Therefore, many young people who are using substances will have a variety of professionals and agencies involved in their care. It may be a teacher who first begins to wonder if a young person's uncharacteristic or unacceptable behaviour is due to substance use. Or it may be a professional working in a family support programme who identifies the need to refer a young person to a specialist substance misuse treatment service. At whatever stage concerns are noticed, it is likely that there will be several adults around the teenager who share those concerns.

Evidence indicates that there are increased benefits for the young person if professionals work in a coordinated fashion. Literature variously describes this as inter-agency, multiagency, interdisciplinary, partnership or collaborative working. The need for inter-agency working may be driven by the fact that a young person is attending several agencies at the same time or by the need for several agencies to pool their resources to provide a service that could not otherwise be provided. Parents and carers are seen as co-colleagues in inter-agency work. This chapter presents the rationale, benefits and challenges of several agencies working together with parents or carers to provide an integrated response to a young person with substance use problems.

RATIONALE FOR INTER-AGENCY WORKING

The benefits of inter-agency collaboration in the care of young people with complex needs have been widely demonstrated.[1-5] Establishing constructive working relationships with children and parents is central to partnership working.[6,7] The majority of teenagers misusing drugs and alcohol do not need child protection services, although some do. However, models that include inter-agency collaboration are particularly suited to working with these teens, as they often experience other difficulties including school refusal, behavioural problems, risk-taking, lawbreaking and loss of hobbies. Young people and families in these contexts are likely to be cared for by several services. For example, a large number of those with substance use problems also have concurrent mental health problems. In addition to substance abuse and mental health services, teens may also be involved with the juvenile justice system or a youth work project while also attending an alternative education setting. The benefits multiply for the teen and his or her family if these services can work coherently and effectively with one another and with the adolescent's family or carers.

Multidimensional Family Therapy (MDFT) is a strongly evidenced systemic treatment model that intentionally engages with the social, educational and family environment of the young person (*see* Chapter 11). The model focuses on relationships with peers, schools and other service providers, with the intention of building relevant supports for the adolescent to prompt change. In the UK, the Common Assessment Framework (CAF) was developed to offer an agreed structure that allowed several agencies working in the area of child protection to quickly and clearly identify the needs of vulnerable children and adolescents. It provides for sharing of information between agencies. Its purpose, as described by Hicks and Stein,[4] is to:

- help to anticipate the additional needs of vulnerable adolescents and children
- enable agencies involved to gain a common understanding of those needs
- develop ways of working together
- indentify a lead agency or practitioner who will be the main contact person with the young person and agencies.

Participating agencies should encourage close working and information sharing. The Munro report affirmed the CAF for client care in local settings but raised concerns that benefits at national level were less clear and identified a risk of it becoming a 'tick box' exercise.[6] The importance of building strong helping relationships with families is therefore vital. The CAF can be adapted to suit a variety of needs. Similar inter-agency agreements can be developed between teams or individual workers who find they are caring for a shared cohort of young people.[1]

VARIATION IN QUALITY AND INTENSITY OF PARTNERSHIP WORKING RELATIONSHIPS

Collaborative advantage and collaborative inertia have been described as two sides of the partnership working coin.[8] Collaborative advantage is gained when something is achieved that could not have been achieved by any organisation working alone. Collaborative inertia is the outcome when very little advantage or progress results from agencies working together. A focused and intentional piece of work is needed to foster good collaboration between agencies, adolescents and carers.

As with interpersonal relationships, there are varying levels of inter-agency relationship.[9] Interpersonal relationships are described in terms of their closeness or distance, their complexity or degree of mutual understanding. To extend the analogy, at one end of the spectrum people can be described as strangers; at the other end, they are described as partners or spouse. In between, there are acquaintances and close friends. Inter-agency relationships tend to operate along a similar spectrum. While agencies strive to build close partnerships, some connections fall short of this ideal. In some cases, there are so many agencies involved with young people with substance misuse problems, it is not possible to have 'true partnership relationships' with them all. Figure 16.1 illustrates the array of services that can be involved. In this case, we can see that

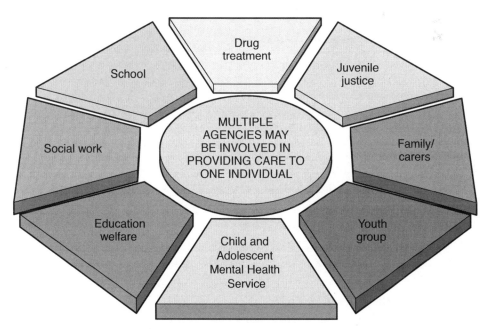

FIGURE 16.1 The complex array of individuals and organisations involved with a teen with substance misuse problems

there are seven other services involved with this young person in addition to the substance misuse service, and this list is by no means exhaustive.

BENEFITS OF INTER-AGENCY WORKING

Inter-agency collaboration can take a variety of forms, such as offering a coordinated treatment approach via a shared care plan, participating in regular multi-agency meetings, making services available to one another's client group or sharing of resources such as premises. In some cases organisations may come together to work jointly for the benefit of one client. For example, staff from a residential care home may work with the substance misuse service to support the client in getting to appointments and support them in carrying out some of the tasks agreed, such as joining a new gym or club. In other instances two services may have many clients in common and so they will probably need to develop a way of working together for all of their clients. Substance misuse services working in conjunction with local mental health services or schools are examples of such collaboration.

BOX 16.1 Ways services can work together

- Involve adolescent and family in collaboration
- Explain inter-agency working, its benefits and gain consent to communicate with other agencies
- Offer a coordinated treatment approach
- Develop a shared plan of care
- Participate in multi-agency meetings for review or information sharing
- Share specialist skills
- Share services and resources

Many benefits accrue if agencies can share information effectively and safely with the client's and family's consent. The need to go through multiple assessments and the need to repeatedly give similar information to each agency can be reduced. Many young people and their families can become frustrated with the duplication of services and the repeated retelling of their story. Lord, *et al.*[1] report one parent's experience of working with agencies using the CAF:

> Although the staff didn't work in the same teams or offices they worked really well together to support us and didn't keep asking us the same questions over and over.

Treatment adherence can be enhanced if the number of appointments in multiple services is reduced. Perhaps a substance misuse treatment service can consider holding its treatment appointments at a juvenile justice service so that the young person achieves both commitments at the same time. If substance misuse services provide treatment in more general youth sites, this may lead to reduced stigma and improve accessibility. This places an onus on other services to provide appropriate rooms to see the clients and other resources as necessary.

BOX 16.2 Reflective practice exercise

- Reflect on current practice in inter-agency working in your service
- What are the pros and cons of your current practice?
- Are there changes that you would like to make?
- Which of these actions are within your remit, capacity and power to do?
- What might the benefits be:
  — for young people?
  — for their families?
  — for your organisation?
  — for you?
- Identify a first step that you can take to benefit your service users

---

There are benefits for agencies as well as young people. Collaborative working reduces duplication and overlap of service provision. Given the need to make best use of resources, several agencies working together can increase efficiencies. All agencies involved in a collaborative piece of work can benefit from the opportunity to learn from professionals working in other settings. This increased awareness of one another's roles enhances practice.

When youth services, schools or juvenile justice services are open to inviting a specialist substance misuse service to conduct sessional work on site, they open up many possibilities for young people. Stigma associated with attending a substance misuse service may be avoided. It can also improve outcomes for clients by making treatment more accessible. It could also increase the likelihood of reluctant young people with drug and alcohol problems engaging in treatment. These initiatives can increase awareness of services in the community and support the up-skilling of staff in identification and management of substance use problems.

Perhaps we have worked too long with the idea that the client must come to our office to engage in a service. While it does create some extra demands on time, it is possible to be flexible in service provision. Creative inter-agency working brings many benefits and can make savings in other ways. The silo mentality of many agencies can be challenged if organisations reflect on their mindset and culture. We can each question taken-for-granted beliefs about how services are provided and make changes that bring benefits for all.

SHARING INFORMATION

How a teenager's information is safeguarded and shared is central to effective collaboration. South Dublin County Council Children's Services Committee describe eight golden rules for sharing information.[10]

1   The safety and welfare of the child is paramount.
2   Openness and honesty about why, with whom, what, where, when and how information may be shared are essential – *unless* doing so creates a risk for safety.
3   Give clear reasons for sharing or requesting consent to share information.
4   Be familiar with your own agency's confidentiality and data protection policies.
5   Data protection legislation provides a framework for appropriate sharing of information.
6   Share with consent, except when getting consent would pose a risk in the situation.
7   Ensure what you share is necessary, timely, relevant, accurate, proportionate and secure. The proportion of information that needs to be shared is decided on the 'need to know' principal.
8   Keep a record of all your decisions, actions and rationale.

The mnemonic NTRAPS emphasises ways to safeguard the information of adolescents and their families (*see* Box 16.3).

BOX 16.3 NTRAPS mnemonic

When sharing information ensure it is:
- Neccessary
- Timely
- Relevant
- Accurate
- Proportionate
- Secure

CHALLENGES TO EFFECTIVE INTER-AGENCY WORKING

As in all relationships the challenges in keeping connections alive, effective and mutually satisfying are many. Challenges to effective inter-agency collaboration include the following.[2,4,11]

- *Lack of trust between agencies*: lack of trust can hamper progress at the initial stages of collaborative working. It may take time and input from all organisations involved to establish a working relationship where all believe that the other agencies are equally committed. Stein[11] reflects on his own experience of inter-agency working; he describes staff from several services having lunch together to foster better working relationships.
- *Different levels of commitment to collaborative work*: commitment can come from either front-line staff or senior management. Without the backup of management the vision to provide a collaborative multi-agency response for young people and families can be hampered, but much can be done even in these circumstances.
- *Lack of understanding, acceptance and mutual respect for the key objectives of each agency*: agencies have different key objectives that need to be balanced – for example, most criminal justice services have the primary goal of keeping the community safe, while health services are primarily focused on the care of the individual young person.
- *Different work practices*: expectations and approaches of team members can be very different, even when dealing with similar situations. This applies all the more to teams from different organisations.
- *Roles of various disciplines*: gaining an understanding of one another's roles can prove challenging. Agencies may struggle to accept the small but inevitable differences of priority or focus that exist between them.
- *Lack of resources to support ongoing collaboration*: good partnership working can bring enormous benefits but it also takes time, effort and investment of staff.
- *Inequalities of power between organisations*: this can lead to struggles between agencies.
- *Concerns about legal issues*: agencies rightly give high priority to issues of confidentiality and consent for the sharing of information related to a young person between agencies. This needs to be constantly revisited and re-evaluated. A young person and his or her family may consent to communication between agencies at a particular time and in relation to specific information. It should not be taken for granted that this applies to all information and all communication. These boundaries need to be thoroughly discussed. As relationships are fostered and built with families and agencies it will become easier to clarify understandings.

Challenges to effective inter-agency working

- Lack of trust between agencies
- Levels of commitment to collaborative work
- Lack of understanding of other objectives
- Different work practices
- Understanding roles of various disciplines
- Lack of resources to support ongoing collaboration
- Inequalities of power between organisations
- Concern about legal issues

ESTABLISHING A PARTNERSHIP INTER-AGENCY AGREEMENT

So, having decided that your agency wants to work collaboratively with others, what's the next step? It's important to plan the manner in which you might develop inter-agency relationships. In our experience, having a policy document or formal agreement is helpful. There is a vast array of information available to help in the development of inter-agency working.[2,4,11] Having an agreed partnership inter-agency agreement (PIA) keeps an intentional focus on the value of working together. This has proved useful to us in noticing who we should be working with and whether we are giving those relationships the attention they require.

Like any relationship, a shared understanding brings depth and breadth to the connection. A PIA provides both agencies a vehicle for describing the delivery of their shared services.[9] It avoids misunderstanding and ensures clarity around service provision, as well as describing the structure upon which that provision rests. The following is one suggested framework for developing such an agreement.

- Identify key agencies that are providing services to teenagers in your area. For example, a school may want to develop inter-agency agreements with mental health or substance misuse services, and vice versa.
- Approach the management of these agencies to seek their cooperation to work jointly, on a pilot basis, in the delivery of a more comprehensive response to meeting the needs of your shared client group.
- Draw up a service agreement with the host agency/s on the principles of a PIA.
- Agree a structure for the delivery of the service. This should clearly state what each agency is required to deliver. For example, the substance use treatment service may agree to attend the second service for 2 hours a week, while the second agency may agree to provide a suitable venue for

the substance misuse professional to meet with young people.

- Agree and document management and reporting structures and feedback mechanisms to ensure the services adapt as needed.
- Audit and evaluate outcomes for young people
- Review and evaluate the effectiveness of the pilot service.

WHAT HELPS INTER-AGENCY PARTNERSHIPS?

Some inter-agency initiatives work well, and we can all learn from what makes these effective. The need for 'moving from compliance to a learning culture' is emphasised.[12] Munro describes the risk of having a legally defensive mind set in delivery of care; the needs of children and families should be central. As professionals, we have an obligation to examine our practice and consider the parts that are less effective. 'Enablers' of inter-agency collaboration have been identified as follows.[2,11]

- *Knowing relevant local services and contact persons within them*: each agency will have built connections with organisations most relevant to their roles. With collaboration comes an extending of the contacts which can lead to increased resources available to adolescents and their families.
- *Trust and respect for the roles and responsibilities of practitioners in other services*: one of the main advantages of inter-agency working is that it allows us to avoid duplication. To achieve this it is vital that we gain a solid understanding of the roles and responsibilities of other professionals. Using a PIA, we can establish who will be doing what with the young person and their family. Clear boundaries are required between the professionals and a genuine respect for each person involved is paramount.
- *Identifying common priorities*: there is risk of becoming entirely focused on one's own agenda. Working on common priorities is beneficial for the young person and their family; however it takes effort and intention to consider what the priorities of other agencies are. Giving them some time and consideration will enrich the working relationship.
- *Clear guidelines and procedures for working together*: clarity around each agency's ways of working will help the partnership. Describing what can be provided by each and how that will be achieved brings clarity. Each will be guided by their own policies and procedures. There may be differences around age of consent for working with adolescents, e.g. some medical practitioners are free to offer treatment to those under 18 years old without parental consent, whereas some organisations cannot. When the practitioners developing the PIA are clear about these differences they

can be disseminated within both organisations; potential struggles may be avoided.

- *Good communication*: including mechanisms for communication between services is vital at the planning stage. Within a PIA, the level of sharing of information that is envisioned can be agreed. If this is clearly laid out, it prevents misunderstanding and promotes collaboration. It is helpful to identify which staff members from which agency will be in communication with each other. The adolescent and their family should also be aware of the agreed level of communication. If needs demand that this changes, it should be discussed further with the young person prior to enacting the change.

- *Regular meetings and contact between meetings*: build in agreed meetings in delivering the PIA. In our work with the juvenile justice service in Ireland, we have developed a strong inter-agency agreement that includes annual meetings with senior management from each service involved. At these meetings, we review the PIA and discuss strengths and limitations of the agreement. In between these meetings, there is regular contact between individual key workers from the substance misuse service and individual probation officers. The important thing to consider when developing the PIA is what form of contact will take place and how often it will occur.

- *Joint training initiatives*: agencies with a common client group will inevitably have some common training needs. Identifying these and fulfilling them together will also help build relationships and is cost-effective. Even if there are different perspectives among organisations, the push and pull of debate in training can lead to better understanding of each other's roles and the development of strong close working ties.[12] It is likely that in some cases one service will be able to provide training to meet the needs of the other organisation.

What helps inter-agency partnerships

- Knowing relevant local services and contact person within them
- Trust and respect
- Identifying common priorities
- Clear guidelines and procedures for working together
- Understanding roles and responsibilities of other practitioners
- Good communication
- Regular meetings
- Joint training initiatives

POSSIBLE STRUCTURE FOR THE DEVELOPMENT OF A PARTNERSHIP INTER-AGENCY RELATIONSHIP

Even if an organisation does not promote engagement with other service providers, one person committed to inter-agency working can bring about change. The benefits of informal as well as formal arrangements for working together have been clearly seen.[2,13] Having given a full explanation of these benefits to the young person and his or her parent or carer, and gained their consent, the practitioner can contact other agencies involved. Simply by letting others know that you are also involved with a young person creates greater coherence for the adolescent.

The PIA is best governed by a written agreement, to be drawn up between the agencies. This agreement should include a management and reporting framework that names the contact person within each agency who will take the lead in ensuring that the close working proceeds in accordance with the agreed framework.

Practical operational issues that will need to be covered in the PIA include:

- the consent and confidentiality guidelines of each agency involved
- how consent to engage with the second service will be obtained from the young person and their guardian
- who carries out the initial assessment
- what services will be provided on what site
- if there are specific service provision needs that should be clarified (e.g. if urine samples are needed as part of a substance misuse treatment model of care, how will this be collected off-site?)
- how files are managed and records are maintained
- who holds ultimate responsibility for the shared care
- the PIA can detail the sharing of facilities, such as what interview rooms might be used, how they will be booked, with whom and what the duration of sessions will be
- agreed protocols for meeting potential challenges to effective inter-agency working; try as far as possible to name difficulties that might arise and name agreed steps for responding to them
- the development of an agreed plan of care for the young person
- an agreed strategy that ensures ongoing monitoring, implementation and evaluation of each client's care
- an agreed strategy for monitoring and evaluating the PIA.

CONCLUSIONS

The skills that increase the quality of inter-agency working are the same skills that ultimately benefit young people and families. Trust building, negotiating, communicating and managing the power imbalances between client and service provider and between one agency and another are needed. Substance misuse problems are often accompanied by an array of other struggles for the adolescent. Inter-agency working guidelines urge parents and workers to ask what it is they do better together that could not be done alone to respond to problems. Focusing on the outcomes helps inter-agency partnerships to keep the needs of the young person and his or her family at the centre. Efficient, effective and ethical inter-agency working smoothes the journey for young people and hopefully hastens the day when they no longer need the services they attend.

KEY POINTS

- Evidence underlines the benefits to adolescents of inter-agency collaboration.
- The adolescent and his or her family or carers are fully partners in that collaboration.
- Information needs to be safeguarded diligently.
- The needs of the adolescent and his or her family are paramount.

FURTHER READING

➡ Munro E. *The Munro Review of Child Protection: interim report; the child's journey.* London: Department for Education; 2011.

➡ *The Common Assessment Framework for children and young people: practitioners' guide.* Available at: www.plymouth.gov.uk/caf_for_practitioners_national_guidance.pdf

REFERENCES

1 Lord P, Kinder K, Wilkin, A, *et al. Evaluating the Early Impact of Integrated Children's Services: Round 1 final report.* Slough: National Foundation for Educational Research; 2008.

2 Children's Act Advisory Board. *Guidance to Support Effective Inter-Agency Work across Irish Children's Services.* Dublin: Children's Act Advisory Board; 2009.

3 Bruns EJ, Walker JS, Zabel M, *et al.* Intervening in the lives of youth with complex behavioural health challenges and their families: the role of the wraparound process. *Am J Community Psychol.* 2010; 46(3–4): 314–31.

4 Hicks L, Stein M. *Neglect Matters: a multi-agency guide for professionals working together on behalf of teenagers.* Nottingham: Department for Children, Schools and Families Publications; 2010. Available at: http://php.york.ac.uk/inst/spru/pubs/1563/ (accessed 9 August 2013).

5 Kelleher K. Organizational capacity to deliver effective treatments for children and adolescents. *Adm Policy Ment Health.* 2010; 37(1–2): 89–94.

6 Munro E. *The Munro Review of Child Protection: Part One. A systems analysis.* London: Department for Education; 2010.

7 Government of Western Australia. *The Signs of Safety Child Protection Practice Framework.* Perth: Child Protection Department, Government of Western Australia: 2011.

8 Vangen S, Huxham C. *Aiming for Collaborative Advantage: challenging the concept of shared vision.* Advanced Institute of Management Research Paper No. 015; 2005. Available at: http://ssrn.com/abstract=1306963 (accessed 11 August 2013).

9 Smyth B. *Guidelines for Interagency Working.* Dublin: Youth Drug & Alcohol Service, Health Service Executive; 2008.

10 South Dublin Children's Services Committee. *Sharing Information about Children and Families: best practice guidelines for practitioners, managers and agencies working in South County Dublin.* Dublin: South Dublin County Council; 2010. Available at: http://children.southdublin.i.e./images/stories/sdcsc_sharing_information.pdf (accessed 11 August 2013).

11 Stein M. *Quality Matters in Children's Services: messages from research.* London: Jessica Kingsley Publishers; 2009.

12 Munro E. *The Munro Review of Child Protection: final report; a child centred system.* London: Department for Education; 2011.

13 Munro E. *The Munro Review of Child Protection: progress report; moving towards a child-centred system.* London: Department for Education; 2012.

CHAPTER 17

Ethical and legal issues

INTRODUCTION

Working with adolescents presents an array of both ethical and legal problems. As discussed in Chapter 4, adolescence is a time of growth and experience. During this time, movement from childhood to adulthood occurs. This change doesn't happen instantly, and so adolescents need to be allowed greater freedom and responsibilities gradually. More important than age is whether the adolescent demonstrates an ability to manage freedom. Therefore, a teenager who always does homework without being reminded may need fewer rules around homework than another teenager who rarely does his or her homework. Most countries restrict children from doing things that may not be in their interest, and allow them to take on board new rights and responsibilities at different ages. The ages at which one can vote, drive, consent to sex and enter into legal contracts are examples of some of these rights. Importantly, the age at which countries give these freedoms varies. For example, most Western countries allow an individual to purchase alcohol at 18 years of age, but in the United States the age is 21 and in Portugal it is 16. Other countries such as Saudi Arabia do not permit the sale of alcohol to anyone. Table 17.1 highlights some of the common rights young people obtain and the ages at which they are obtained in different countries.

The variation can largely be explained on cultural grounds. The laws of each country generally reflect the attitudes and beliefs of the majority of its citizens. These beliefs and attitudes can be based on historical traditions and religious beliefs. For example, predominantly Muslim countries tend to have stricter laws on alcohol use. Bearing all of that in mind, working with teenagers throws up a considerable number of dilemmas. Substance-using teens can break the law by having a substance in their possession. Likewise, they are more likely to engage in risky sexual behaviours and to be at increased risk from a child protection perspective. These risks create minefields for practitioners working

TABLE 17.1 Overview of ages at which young people obtain various rights

Activities	Country
Consent to sex	
13	Spain (due to be raised to 16 in 2013)
14	Italy, Hungary, Croatia
15	France, Denmark
16	UK, Netherlands
17	Ireland
14–18	United States, depending on state and gender
16–18	Australia, depending on state
	Note that in many countries ages vary depending on states/regions, gender, and for homosexual and heterosexual sex. Homosexual acts are illegal in some countries.
Vote in elections	
16	Jersey
18	Ireland, UK, United States, France, New Zealand, Australia
20	Japan
	EU laws only allow those over 18 to vote in EU elections. Austria allows 16-year-olds to vote in local and national elections but they cannot vote in EU elections. Almost all countries allow voting from 18 years of age, but some have restrictions on gender and some differentiate between different elections.
Purchasing alcohol	
16	Portugal, Italy
18	UK, Ireland, New Zealand, Australia, Spain
21	United States
	Some countries have different ages for purchasing and consuming alcohol. Others, such as Belgium, Germany and some areas of Austria, have different ages for buying beer (16 years) and spirits (18 years).
	Many Islamic counties prohibit alcohol sale and consumption.

Note: EU, European Union

with adolescents, and much of the time there are no clear and simple answers. Frequently, the law and ethics may appear to be at odds with each other. In order to provide some guidance in this area, some common legal and ethical dilemmas will be explored in this chapter.

Making decisions on complex ethical dilemmas is not easy, and many theories have been suggested that can help. Four key ethical principles repeatedly appear in healthcare literature to provide a framework for practitioners. These are summarised in Box 17.1. While on the surface they appear simple, they regularly come into conflict with each other. For example, should a 16-year-old be allowed to continue to use heroin if he or she wishes (autonomy) or should the 16-year-old be placed in secure care to be protected from him- or herself (beneficence)?

BOX 17.1 The four key ethical principles

1 *Autonomy* suggests that individuals have the right to make their own decisions and to determine what is best for themselves.
2 *Beneficence* suggests that practitioners should act in the best interest of the client.
3 *Non-maleficence* requires the practitioner to do nothing that will cause harm to the client.
4 *Justice* requires practitioners to treat all clients equally.

Note: Adapted from Charles-Edwards and Glasper[1]

Besides ethical principles, practitioners need to be aware of the responsibilities placed on them legally by the state or country they are in, as well as by their own professional organisation and employer. Ignoring ethical and legal obligations can have serious consequences including criminal prosecution, being sued, fired and professional disbarment. When making decisions that are ethically challenging we suggest the following steps.

- Avoid making quick decisions – complex decisions deserve time to be considered fully.
- Do not make decisions alone – discuss them with colleagues, managers and supervisors.
- Document clearly the decision made, the rationale for the decision and any steps in making the decision, such as discussions with others.

DILEMMA 1: ABSTINENCE VERSUS CONTROLLED USE

Case Study 1

Bill is 16 years old and drinks alcohol almost daily – usually about eight 500 mL cans of lager. He recognises that his drinking is causing harm, particularly in getting him in trouble with the police. He has numerous charges for public order offences and wants to avoid further trouble. However, he states clearly that he does not want to stop drinking, despite the fact that the legal drinking age is 18. Instead, he wants to drink on weekends only, which he sees as normal for boys his age.

Most people believe that when adolescents misuse a drug or alcohol, it would be much better if they stopped. However, some people take this idea further and believe that they *must* stop, and so only abstinence is a suitable goal. Some argue that if you do not work with the teen to stop the drug use, you are colluding with them and giving the message that it's okay for him or her to continue using. On the surface, this appears to make sense, but further analysis raises a few important issues, outlined here.

- In reality, a significant proportion of teens use drugs and alcohol, with only a minority of these coming for treatment. Most will simply grow out of problematic drug and alcohol use, giving it up of their own accord.
- Many of the teens who use drugs do not believe they have a problem. If they come for treatment, it is frequently because someone has put pressure on them to do so. If they do not want to stop using, they are unlikely to work at stopping. However, it might be possible to help them recognise that the amount or frequency of their use is problematic. That recognition may lead them to reduce their use significantly.
- As outlined in Chapter 9, motivation is usually diminished when people believe they are being forced to accept something they do not agree with. Simply insisting that teenagers stop using is rarely helpful. Usually, the conversation goes nowhere and the teenager disengages. It is consequently more than unhelpful to try to force a client to be abstinent – in fact, it may even be harmful!
- The majority of teenagers who use substances use more than one. They may smoke cannabis and drink, for example. Even if you get them to stop one substance they may not stop the other.

The importance of listening to the young person's views cannot be overstated. Bordin[2] proposed a useful way for conceptualising the relationship between a client and a professional. He suggests three vital components to a working or therapeutic alliance: (1) bonds, (2) tasks and (3) goals. 'Bonds' refers to the relationship between the client and practitioner. If a client does not believe the professional can help him or her, or does not trust the professional, it is unlikely he or she will engage meaningfully, and so progress will be difficult. Likewise, the client will only work on a 'goal' that he or she sees as worth working on. Finally, if a client is to achieve the goal, he or she will need to agree with the practitioner about what 'tasks' need to be done to achieve it.

If we apply Bordin's idea to the 'abstinence versus controlled' debate we can see that when the practitioner insists on a goal the client does not subscribe to, the practitioner is unlikely to engage the client. The client will probably become frustrated and disengage, resulting in even poorer outcomes. Alternatively, the practitioner who accepts the client's goal of controlled or reduced use, even if the practitioner does not believe it to be a good idea, is likely to improve the working relationship with the client. If the practitioner succeeds in helping the client reduce his or her use and associated harm, the practitioner has attained some success. Also, if the controlled plan does not work, while the client is engaged in a process of dealing with his or her use, the client may then decide that a period of abstinence is worth trying. Neither of these outcomes is likely if the client has dropped out of therapy. It is also worth noting that accepting a person's goal is not the same as agreeing with it. We frequently tell clients that we would prefer them to stop using but that if they are determined to continue use we would like to help them to ensure they suffer the least amount of harm as a result.

There are ways other than abstinence of measuring success. One option is to measure the client's substance use in terms of frequency, duration and intensity.[3] A client who does not stop using a substance can make considerable changes in any of these three areas. For example, a client who drinks may spend fewer days drinking (frequency), shorten the time of drinking episodes (duration), or drink less alcohol when drinking (intensity). All these changes, while short of abstinence, are quantifiable improvements and steps in the right direction. Likewise, improved relationships with family, improved attendance in education and better health are also valid measures of success.

Arguably, while it is admirable to want to do as much as possible for a substance-using adolescent, one must accept reality. Not everyone will want to become abstinent. If you can help some make the decision to stop, brilliant. However, for the many other clients who refuse to stop, any reduction in harm is an improvement. The last thing you want is to be so insistent on abstinence that you effect no change where you could have actually made a real difference. It is hardly ethical to force your opinions on a client to the client's detriment.

DILEMMA 2: REPORTING RISKY BEHAVIOURS TO CHILD PROTECTION SERVICES

Case Study 2

Angela is 15 years old and has been brought to a substance misuse service by her parents. Angela reports using a variety of substances including cannabis, alcohol, ecstasy and benzodiazepines. She rarely goes a day without using some drugs and admits her life is not going well. She is doing poorly in school, has dropped out of her hobbies and frequently does not come home at night. She is tearful and wants to change.

If you work with clients who use substances, you will invariably identify risky behaviours. These may include the drug use itself, but also associated behaviours such as having sex, criminality, and so forth. As a practitioner, you will be faced with a dilemma: do you report the behaviour to the appropriate person such as a social worker or not? Naturally, this is more relevant when working with teenagers than adults due to the onus on professionals to protect children who are inherently vulnerable. The case for reporting to a social worker can be argued either way.

- *For*
  - Referral to a social worker ensures the teenager is protected and given all the resources available to help them.
  - It ensures that the practitioner is covered – they have done all they can.
- *Against*
  - Reporting a young person or family at risk to social workers may not be welcomed by them, and it may lead to damage in the therapeutic alliance between them and the reporting service.
  - If the public view a service as very likely to report them to a social worker, they may be less likely to approach that service for help. This can affect the service's ability to work with other families at risk, and it can influence whether or not families will be honest when they do engage.

Rather than focusing on past risks the teenager has engaged in, it is more useful to look at the trajectory of risk. When there is real and immediate risk to the young person, it is necessary to get relevant professionals involved. This can happen in cases of suicidality or ongoing physical or sexual abuse. However, in most cases, substance use itself rarely brings such obvious immediate risks and, in these instances, the trajectory the client is on is vital. A client who, like Angela in Case Study 2, engages and wants to make changes, could be allowed the opportunity to make these changes without reporting, as risks will be declining. On the other hand, if Angela were to drop out, not make progress, or increase her risky behaviour (say, by starting to use heroin), then it makes sense to report in light of the increasing risks.

DILEMMA 3: INVOLVING PARENTS (OR NOT!)

Case Study 3

Dexter is 15 years old and presents at a substance use service asking for help with his drug use. He has been smoking cannabis daily for about a year. He never really knew his father, and he lives with his mother and stepfather. He does not get on well with them and does not think they know about his cannabis use and does not want them to know. Dexter believes telling them would simply lead to more problems at home. He wants to come for treatment on condition that they are not informed – if his parents have to be told, he will not come to treatment.

Getting parents involved in the treatment of their teens' substance use is very important. There is considerable evidence demonstrating positive benefit for teens when their parents are involved. Most evidence-based treatments for adolescent substance abuse, such as Multidimensional Family Therapy and the Adolescent Community Reinforcement Approach, have strong parenting components (*see* Chapter 8). Research repeatedly demonstrates that parenting practices are influential on adolescent substance use. Thus, having parents involved in treatment should be the goal.

So, once we accept that it is preferable to have the parents involved, the situation will sometimes arise where a teenager refuses to allow their involvement, and this can happen in a variety of ways. The teenager may wish to attend a service without his or her parents' knowledge, or the teenager may try to disrupt the level of involvement his or her parents have – for example, by refusing to sit in sessions with them. Even if the teen completely refuses to engage, working with the parents without the teen in the room can be very effective, and we cannot make a young person sit in a session. If the teen refuses to sit in sessions with his or her parents, work can be done with the teen and parents separately. They can always be brought together later if the situation improves between them.

The amount of information shared with parents can also be difficult to negotiate. While parents may realise their child is using drugs, they may not know all the details and their teenager may not want them to know. Teens may ask that certain information such as what drugs they have used, how frequently they used them, or other behaviours related to drug use are kept from their parents. On the one hand, it is good to encourage open communication between the parent and teen, but the most important thing is the long-term outcome for the child. A useful approach is to have a standard agreement with parents and teens that what is discussed in the individual sessions is kept between the counsellor and the teen, assuring both that confidentiality will have to be broken where there is escalating risks or immediate risk of harm to someone. Hence, if the teen's drug use is getting worse or if they are suicidal, then we may have to talk to parents and the teen is supported to join in this conversation. Most parents are happy that their child is talking to someone, and so this rarely causes problems. In general, we would encourage the teen to allow some feedback on what is being worked on to the parents. If concerns persist, it is important that you try to maintain the working relationship with the teen. One of the best ways of doing this is by helping the teen discuss things with his or her parents, rather than the practitioner doing it on the teen's behalf.

In rare cases, a teenager may present for treatment for a substance use problem on his or her own and ask that parents are not involved or informed. This raises the question of whether or not teenagers can consent to treatment. Some services also require that both parents consent to treatment. As many teenagers are not very motivated to stop their drug use, we believe in making services as user-friendly and accessible as possible. The age at which a young person can consent to treatments varies from country to country, and in many cases it is not very clear. For example, in Ireland the law states that once past your sixteenth birthday you are allowed to consent on your own to 'medical, surgical and dental treatments'.[4] It seems logical that if you are deemed competent to consent to surgery, surely you are competent to consent to counselling. Hence, as this is not stated within the relevant act, it is a grey area. In the UK, a landmark case essentially did away with the idea of a set age for consenting, and, instead, said that a child who was competent to consent could do so and essentially be treated as an adult for the purposes of medical treatment.[5] Some have argued that this is not a satisfactory situation, as the practitioner has to decide who is competent.[6] Many readers may feel that if they are not treating the substance use problem, the issue of consent is not relevant to them. However, schools or youth services need their own policy about how they can refer a teen for appropriate treatment. Is it okay for a teacher to refer a 15- or 16-year-old student to a substance abuse service without informing the parents or guardians?

In the end when working with substance-using teens we suggest the following.

- As a general rule, get parents involved.
- Ensure the teen is seen alone and that he or she is given time to speak openly.
- Manage secrets sensibly – teens cannot be expected to tell their parents everything, but neither should they be allowed to keep secrets that place themselves or others at risk.
- In the rare cases when teens refuse to allow their parents be involved, we suggest that services should allow for the young person to be referred for treatment and allow the specialist service to make a call on competence to consent.
- If seeing adolescents in relation to their substance use without parental consent, each practitioner will have to make a judgement call. In these situations it is important to not make decisions alone, avail of supervision and be mindful of specific laws and policies in your country and organisation.

DILEMMA 4: REPORTING CRIMINAL ACTIVITIES

Case Study 4

Mary is 17 years old. She is attending a substance abuse service for her alcohol use following referral from her school. During the assessment, Mary speaks openly about being involved in a variety of criminal activities. She admits to regularly 'shoplifting' various items – typically alcohol, but also clothes and CDs. She also gets in physical fights with people when drunk. She knows that at least one person she fought ended up in hospital for a few days, but this person seems fine now. These fights happen every 2–3 weeks. Mary has never been arrested or charged with any crimes.

Teenagers who use drugs and alcohol can break the law in a number of ways. Depending on their age and the country they are in, using drugs or alcohol alone may be illegal. Likewise, *where* they use can be a crime – in many countries it is illegal to drink in public areas such as streets or parks. In order to fund their substance use, they may also be involved in shoplifting, robbery and other crime. Sometimes, drug users present with extreme antisocial behaviours such as aggression and violence (often in the family home), stealing cars, vandalism, breaking into houses and other properties.

Asking about criminal and risky behaviours allows for a full assessment, but presents you with a question of what to do with the information you uncover. On the other hand, not asking means you aren't getting true insight to the level of risk for this young person, and so are unlikely to be able to deal with it appropriately. This option is appealing, as it lets you off the hook as you have nothing to report.

There is an ethical obligation on professionals to do a thorough assessment in order to provide appropriate interventions. Putting your head in the sand means you are unlikely to be responding appropriately. If you uncover criminal behaviour, we believe there is only an obligation on the practitioner to report when there is a real and clear risk to the client or someone else. It is not the role of the practitioner to ensure his or her clients are prosecuted to the full extent of the law for every legal infringement. Reporting past crimes will not change what has been done. More important, if clients believe their past behaviours will be reported, they will not be honest. Such a situation is hardly conducive to change.

A caveat should be added here in relation to information regarding sexual assault or child abuse. If a client reports sexually assaulting someone in the past, or sexually abusing children, the local child protection guidelines should be adhered to. Most countries have national policies on reporting incidents of reported sexual abuse or assault.

DILEMMA 5: DRUG DEALING AND DRUG DEBTS

Case Study 5

Fred is a 16-year-old school student. He began smoking cannabis at 13 and he has been smoking daily for about a year and a half. Typically, the value of the cannabis he smokes is €200–€300 every week. He has never used any other drug and does not intend to. For the past year, he has funded this by selling cannabis to other students in his school. He generally makes enough to pay for his own use, but on two occasions recently he could not repay a debt to another dealer. In return for the dealer wiping these debts, Fred agreed to store cocaine. Fred estimates that the cocaine was worth about €2000.

One of the most complicated and challenging situations we have encountered over the past few years is drug dealing and debts. Take a moment to understand how this can happen for a fairly typical teenager. Once a teenager commences drug use – say, cannabis, which is the most commonly used drug – he or she needs to find a way to pay for it. Depending on the drug and level of use, this can be expensive. In adolescent cannabis smokers, the amount used can vary widely, ranging from a €50 bag between a few friends once a week to smoking a €50 bag each every day – this amounts to about €350 per week, which is a huge sum of money. Clearly, this level of use does not happen overnight.

Typically, teenagers start off smoking a few joints here or there. In most instances, their first use involves sharing a friend's joint. Gradually, they may want to use more frequently and start to buy their own. Soon, the cannabis they buy is lasting less and less time. Over a few months, they begin to smoke more frequently. This is similar to the manner in which teenagers start smoking cigarettes. Obviously, this increased use is more expensive. Once a connection to a dealer is established, the adolescent may become an access to cannabis for his or her friends. When the adolescent goes to the dealer with a bigger order (for him- or herself and friends), he or she gets better deals and discounts. As the adolescent is passing cannabis on to friends, he or she is now effectively dealing. Before long, the adolescent gets known as someone who has access, and so he or she is dealing more and more.

This happens gradually and so many teens do not see it as dealing – in their eyes, they are simply helping their friends get cannabis. To them, it is similar to an adult picking up some beer for a friend on the way to a party. One of the dangers with dealing is that it regularly operates on a credit system. A teen gets hold of, say, €300 worth of cannabis on credit, which he divides into eight €50 bags. He plans to sell six of the bags to recoup the €300 to pay off the debt, leaving two bags for his own use at no cost. However, things may not go according to plan. The adolescent ends up using more than he intended, his friends fail to come up with money they promised, or the cannabis gets confiscated by his parents or the police. As a result, he is left with the debt and no means to pay it.

Commonly, this is when things come to a head. The teenager has come home fearful for his safety, as a dealer is demanding payment for a debt. The threat isn't always just hanging over the teen, but also his family. Parents frequently pay the debt to keep their child safe. In many cases, they have paid numerous debts and are borrowing significant sums of money. This creates a dangerous situation. The teen learns that if he messes up and runs up drug debts, his parents will pay, so long as they are concerned for the teen's safety. What is the incentive for him to stop? The teen also gets a reputation of being a reliable payer, perhaps improving his credit rating with dealers.

When working with such families we are frequently asked by the parents, 'what should I do? Should I pay?' The simple answer is no, because the teenager needs to learn that this behaviour is not acceptable. They have to become uncomfortable enough with the situation for them to be bothered to change. This is easy for us to say, it is not our child. We are not the ones who will be up at night worrying. In reality, we cannot make this decision for parents, we cannot tell them what to do. It is a situation where the end result is unclear. In reality, teenagers are beaten or hurt, sometimes seriously, over drug debts. Naturally, the level of risk may vary from country to country. No professional wants to tell a parent to not pay a debt and then discover that the teen is seriously hurt or killed as a result. As well as having such an outcome on your conscience, it may also leave you open to legal action. When working with these parents, we recommend the following.

- Help the parent understand how this can happen – humanise the teen and their situation.
- Discuss in an open, unhurried and calm manner the pros and cons of both paying and not paying. Explore the possible and likely outcomes of each scenario.
- Reflect on a third option of contacting the police.
- Explain clearly the reasons why you cannot make this decision for them.
- Support the parents with whatever decision they come to, and help them re-evaluate their decision in the future if necessary.
- Explore other steps that can be taken so that the consequences of their actions are understood by the teen.

CONCLUSION

As demonstrated by the discussions in this chapter, substance use creates many complicated and challenging scenarios. Many have no clear or simple answers. A serious problem requires serious deliberation. Discussing it with colleagues or a supervisor is helpful. Check for any laws, policies or guidelines that may help you make the decision. Finally, document clearly the decision you make, the rationale for this decision and the process of deliberation you went through to arrive at the decision, such as whom you discussed it with or policies you examined.

KEY POINTS

- Adolescents who are using drugs tend to present with various behaviours and problems that trigger ethical and legal dilemmas.
- These dilemmas can make dealing with teenage substance use problems stressful.
- In most cases dilemmas do not have to be dealt with straight away and so it is advisable for staff to take the opportunity to discuss them with colleagues, line managers and supervisors.
- Local and national policies need to be taken into account and so practitioners are advised to familiarise themselves with these policies.
- Having well-thought-out policies help in dealing with such situations and as situations arise they feed into the development and updating of policies.

FURTHER READING

- The AVERT website provides information on the legal age of consent to sexual activities for most countries (www.avert.org/age-of-consent.htm).
- *Sexual health*: sexual activities among teenagers can raise many legal and ethical questions. Chapter 14 in this book provides more information on this topic. Further information is also available in Sarah Bekaert's book (Bekaert S. *Adolescents and Sex: the handbook for professionals working with young people*. Oxford: Radcliffe Publishing; 2005).
- *Developing policies*: this chapter also highlights the need for having clear policies in place to guide how situations are dealt with. Chapter 12 in this book provides further information on developing policies within schools and other youth organisations.

REFERENCES

1 Charles-Edwards I, Glasper EA. Ethics and children's rights: learning from past mistakes. *Br J Nurs*. 2002; **11**(17): 1132–40.

2 Bordin ES. The generalisability of the psychoanalytic concept of the working alliance. *Psychother Theor Res.* 1979; **16**(3): 252–60.

3 Bishop FM. *Managing Addictions: cognitive, emotive, and behavioral techniques.* Northvale, NJ: Jason Aronson; 2001.

4 Government of Ireland. *Non-Fatal Offences Against the Person Act.* Dublin: The Stationery Office; 1997.

5 Gillick v West Norfolk and Wisbech Health Authority. [1986] AC112.

6 Hunter D, Pierscionek PK. Children, Gillick competency and consent for involvement in research. *J Med Ethics.* 2007; **33**(11): 659–62.

Index

Entries in **bold** denote figures, tables and boxes.

12-step approach 179–82, 195
'3-S Philosophy' 182

AA (Alcoholics Anonymous) 109, 119,
  179–82, 195
abscesses 36, 45, 48, 52, 63
abstinence
  for adolescents 81, 125–6, 264–5
  and heroin overdose 44
  rewards for 185, 192
acamprosate 191
accidents 26, 39, 41, 48, 57–8, 68–9
ACRA (Adolescent Community
  Reinforcement Approach)
  elements for parents 137–8
  and harm reduction 125
  and operant conditioning 163–4
  procedures of 164–5, 168–71,
    173–4
  substance use in 161–2
  training in 175
addicted self 123, 182
addiction
  disease model of 119–20, **120–1**
  in ICD-10 118
  neurobiological basis of 60
  use of term 3–4
addiction services 55, 116–17
addictiveness 37
ADHD (attention deficit hyperactivity
  disorder) 85–6, 214–15, 221
adolescence
  brain change during 15
  cultural diversity of 9–10
  developmental stages of 20, 201
  and sex 225–6
  stereotypes of **10–11**, 11–12, 26–7
  use of term 5
adolescent substance use
  and anxiety 216–17
  consequences of 1
  and development 57

diagnosing 117–19
differences from adults **122–3**
effects on others 200
ethical dilemmas over 263–8, 272
evidence-based models of 137
features of 6–7
and health promotion **95**
intervention in 110
parents dealing with 135
preventing 93–4
risks of 68–9
screening for 112–13
services responding to 113–15
social attitudes to 201–2
surveys of 91, **92**
treatment of 121, 123–4, 185, 189–90,
  195
adolescents, *see* teenagers
adults, influence of 77–8
affirmation 152
age, and competence 29–30
agencies, key objectives of 253
AIDS 231
alcohol 37–8
  and accidental injury 58–9
  classification of 34
  delaying onset of use 66–7, 81, 201
  as drug 111
  and dual diagnosis 210
  effects of 38–9, 59–60, 63
  and fun 66–7
  as gateway drug 60–1, 69, 92–3
  and gender 240–1
  legal age of use 261, 263
  low-risk use of **38**
  onset of use 79, 81
  parental provision of 79–80, 89, 96
  pharmacology of 35, 37
  prevalence of use **40**
  promotion of 103–4
  and religion 241
  risks of use 39

CPD with Radcliffe

You can now use a selection of our books to achieve CPD (Continuing Professional Development) points through directed reading.

We provide a free online form and downloadable certificate for your appraisal portfolio. Look for the CPD logo and register with us at: www.radcliffehealth.com/cpd

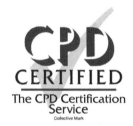